DON'T LET YOUR

HMO

KILL YOU

DON'T LET YOUR
HMO
KILL YOU

HOW TO WAKE UP YOUR DOCTOR,
TAKE CONTROL OF YOUR HEALTH,
AND MAKE MANAGED CARE WORK FOR YOU

JASON THEODOSAKIS, MD, MS, MPH
AND
DAVID T. FEINBERG, MD

ROUTLEDGE
New York & London

9997560

Published in 2000 by
Routledge
29 West 35th Street
New York, NY 10001

Published in Great Britain by
Routledge
11 New Fetter Lane
London EC4P 4EE

Copyright © 2000 by Routledge

Printed in the United States of America on acid-free paper
Design: Jack Donner

While every attempt has been made to make all of the information in this book as accurate and up to date as possible, conditions, medications, and human knowledge change. Before making a final decision on any substantive matter covered in this book, you should seek the advice of an appropriate professional.

Some of the product names, trademarks, and descriptive names used in this publication are registered trademarks, proprietary names, registered designs, etc., even though they may not be specifically designated as such. This does not mean that such names, as described in the Trade Marks and Merchandise Marks Act, are in the public domain.

To protect and respect the privacy of those who have shared their stories with us, all identifying information of real persons described in this book has been altered.

Library of Congress Cataloging-in-Publication Data

Theodosakis, Jason.
    Don't let your HMO kill you: how to wake up your doctor, take control of your health, and make managed care work for you / by Jason Theodosakis and David T. Feinberg.
        p.   cm.
    ISBN 0-415-92482-0 (pb.)
    1. Health maintenance organizations—United States Popular works. 2. Managed care plans (Medical care)—United States Popular works. 3. Consumer education. I. Feinberg, David T. II. Title.
    RA413.5.U5T48   1999
    362.1'04258—dc21   99-35006
                                                            CIP

Since we are both the only doctors in our families,
we get many medical and managed care questions
from aunts, uncles, cousins, and in-laws.
When selecting the advice to give in this book,
we thought about the advice we have given them.
We hope the lessons we have learned serve your family
as well as they have served ours.

We dedicate this book to our families.

~

Contents

~ 1 ~
The Managed Care Nightmare

QUESTIONS THIS CHAPTER ANSWERS

◆ *Why is my doctor so rushed?*

◆ *Why do I get only ten minutes with my doctor?*

◆ *Where do my premiums go?*

◆ *What's wrong with old-fashioned health care?*

◆ *How can this book help me?*

If something like this has never happened to you, count yourself lucky. You show up for your appointment on time. With a smile, you greet the receptionist sitting behind a generic white countertop. It's then that you know something is wrong. Barely moving her gaze from the computer terminal, she motions with her hand to an open notebook. "Sign in there," she commands.

You notice then that there are a dozen names already on the sheet, and the ink is still fresh. You turn to the waiting room. It's packed. One woman listlessly leafs through a two-month-old issue of *Time*. A man nervously looks at his watch, leans back, and then looks again. A child runs through the rows of unpadded seats, unsupervised by his father, who seems to be fast asleep. An elderly man sits in the farthest corner, coughing. This is going to be a long wait, and none too pleasant.

You are due back at work in an hour. You try to expedite your visit by asking the receptionist if you can settle your co-payment now, while you are waiting, instead of after you see the doctor. She points to a sign: "Please pay in full before you leave." That doesn't really answer your question, but you decide not to start a fight. "After you sign in," she drones, "fill out this form."

The form has the same questions you have been asked a dozen times before, but you dutifully answer questions about your past medical history. Then you wait. And wait. Your name is finally called.

You are herded into an examining room, told to strip, and left alone. Then you wait. And wait. That two-month old issue of *Time* is starting to look entertaining compared to the biohazard warning on a disposal bin that you read as you wait. And wait.

When the door finally opens, your anger and frustration has built to the point where you want to lash out at the doctor. He's not helping. He's obviously impatient as you describe your problem, clearly dismissive as you express your concern. As you leave, preparing yourself for another rude encounter with the receptionist, you wonder: "Did we institute socialized medicine and did someone just forget to tell me? Was I just put on welfare and sent to a county hospital? Aren't I paying good money for health insurance? What happened to that smiling, good-looking doctor on my brochure?"

It's not quite socialized medicine, and it's not the county hospital. It's managed care, and in case you haven't heard, it's the way things are for nearly every American who has health insurance. It happened so quickly that virtually no one, not even the vast majority of doctors, has fully come to grips with the realities and pitfalls of the new system. How quickly did this revolution turn health care around? In 1984, only 15 million Americans were enrolled in a managed care program. Ninety-five percent of those enrolled in a company health plan were in a traditional indemnity plan, whereby the patient could see any doctor, and rarely saw a bill. In 1999, an estimated 83 percent of insured employees were in managed care. Employees still insured by indemnity made up the rest—a mere 17 percent.

It happened way too fast for most of us. We continue to hold onto our old-fashioned ideas about doctors and hospitals—about the welcome mats they placed at their doorsteps, about how the patient was first and the bill was second, about how the best care in the world should be available on demand. Managed care was careful to not let us know that they were changing all that. Their advertisements and brochures assured us that everything was going to be fine.

Now we know that's all a lie, and most of us are furious. But what

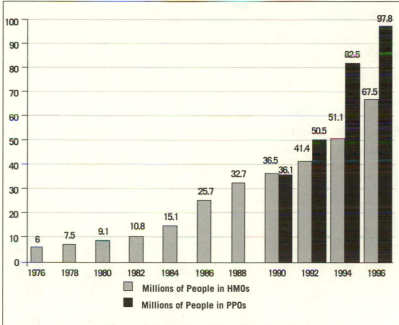

Figure 1.1 Managed Care Enrollment
Source: American Association of Health Plans

In 1976, federal funding for HMOs encouraged development of the new system, but the new plans didn't draw many customers. Migration to managed care began to accelerate in the late eighties as employers faced premium increases of as much as 20 percent a year. PPOs moved quickly to offer managed care with the option of choosing doctors from a list, and now are serious competition to the "traditional" HMO models.

can we do? Few of us can switch managed care companies like we would switch brands of a consumer product. Few of us can take the time to figure out how this new system works. Hardly anyone can make sense of the alphabet soup of health plans we are swimming in today. We've got HMO, MBHO, IPA, PHO, MSO, PPO, EPO, POS, PPM, or IDS. But any way you arrange these letters, they spell one thing: madness.

This book is going to cut to the chase. Instead of taking you through all the intricacies of each plan and each possible plan, this guide will focus on the questions most important to you, the consumer of health care:

- How can I get the best treatment?
- How can I make my HMO listen to my needs?
- How can I improve my relationship with my doctor?
- How can I make the most of every visit?

These questions will take time to answer, but one very important tip will get you started. Unless you are an active rather than a passive patient, you will never get the care you deserve. Unless you are prepared to stand up for your rights, your HMO will someday let you down.

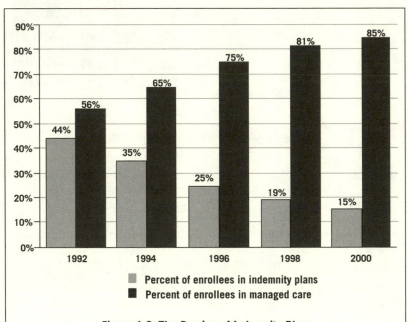

Figure 1.2 The Demise of Indemnity Plans
Source: The Lewin Group

Traditional indemnity insurance has all but disappeared with the rise of the managed care organizations. Ninety percent of doctors these days have at least one managed care contract. And since indemnity insurance is so rare, those few who have it now must pay even more inflated premiums as doctors charge those patients even higher rates. This is known as "cost-shifting," and will accelerate the final end of indemnity insurance for all but the wealthiest consumers.

You might not become a statistic or a sensational headline, but at some stage, your managed care plan's need to make money will come in conflict with your need to be listened to, cared for, and treated. It happens in small and subtle ways as well as dramatic ways. It happened to one of our friends. We'll call her Mara, and let her story illustrate the biggest single problem with managed care—the loss of quality time with your doctor.

We'll then look at what sort of treatment she might have gotten in the old fee-for-service system, explain why those days are gone, and explain why we shouldn't miss them. This is important to understand because your doctor is confronted with this reality daily, and understanding your doctor is the key to getting proper care.

Mara's Story—The Ten-Minute Visit

No one is immune from a system that puts intense financial pressures on doctors. Mara found that out when she went into her HMO for an annual "well woman" visit, which is a simple pelvic exam and pap smear by an OB-GYN. Mara isn't a typical patient—she's a doctor who keeps up with the latest developments in medicine—but her experience is all too typical.

"It was my first visit to this doctor," she told us, "and I noticed that everything was hurried. I get into the table and I'm in the stirrups while he's doing the exam, and I'm trying to ask him a few questions. Being a young, single woman in the nineties, I thought maybe I should get screened for HIV, and I wanted to ask him about that. And I had an ongoing question about irregular periods that I wanted to ask him about, too. But he stopped me before I even got the words out. He just held up his hand and said, "This is a well-woman visit and you're not supposed to have any questions. We're only allowed ten minutes per patient."

Ten minutes per patient. Who sets this rule? What difference does it make? And why would a doctor not want Mara's information and questions? We'll address these questions soon, but first let's see what happened to Mara. "There I am in the stirrups and he won't even take a minute to answer a question!" she continues. "I was so shocked that I didn't press him. He said, 'You have to make another appointment if you want to ask questions.' I wanted to get up and run out of the room, but of course I was in no position to do that. So, feeling as though I'd been treated like a child, I just did what I was told and made another appointment."

Many patients would have given up at this point. Maybe that's what some HMOs are hoping for. But Mara was determined to get the most out of her health plan and took yet more time off from work for another try. "I got an appointment with a woman this time," she says, "and once I got there, I found out that she wasn't a doctor but a nurse practitioner. I'm trying to be responsible and take care of myself, so I started asking her all my questions about sexually transmitted diseases. I also said, again, that I wanted to get screened for HIV. At that point, she advised me not to get tested there because if I were to have an HIV test in my records, she said the HMO might look at that and it would somehow count against me. So she pulled out a stack of cards from Planned Parenthood and gave me one and told me that I could go there anonymously and get the test for free."

Mara says the whole experience left a bitter taste in her mouth: "I keep thinking, I'm a doctor, but I still felt powerless to question what they were doing, even though it was infuriating. I'm really busy, and I didn't feel I had the time to fight it. And the nurse scared me about the confidentiality of the test I wanted." This distrust came from only two encounters, and even though Mara didn't lose a leg or have her life threatened by bureaucratic incompetence, the system let her down in almost every way. She got nothing from her visit but a Pap smear. She won't even know the results of the test unless she asks—even if it's abnormal. Although she is a doctor herself, in a position to speak to her gynecologist as an equal, she was humiliated by the situation in his office. What happened?

Why Is My Doctor So Rushed?

Mara's story gives us clues to what is wrong with managed care, but we have to look behind the cold reactions of the doctor and the dismissal of the nurse practitioner to see what made them act the way they did. In truth, they were trained as caregivers, and perhaps never expected that they would have to be so abrupt with their patients. In truth, it's all about money.

"We're allowed only ten minutes per patient."

Mara saw this as an outrageous statement with only one purpose—to give her the brush-off. But there are reasons behind this rudeness. Managed care is, and always will be, a volume business. Mara is in what is called a "capitated plan." That means that the HMO gets a flat rate for covering a group of customers for a set period, whether they come in or not. So there is a real benefit in keeping her out of the doctor's office. If she does come in for a routine visit, there's a real benefit in moving her out the door as quickly as possible, so another patient can take her place. The doctor Mara saw might work on a salary, or he might work on a per-patient basis. Either way, the managed care organization will offer him incentives to keep costs down. Either way, he will be rewarded for moving Mara down the assembly line as quickly as possible.

Allotting ten minutes per patient isn't a way for him to get to the golf course on time. It's a survival mechanism. These days, it's hard for even the best doctors to survive in private practice. On his first day, he might have walked into the clinic with a spring in his step and taken his time with each patient, putting her at ease and explaining each procedure. But by the end of the day, he's four or five patients behind.

As the waiting room fills, patients begin to grumble, some walk out, and some might even call their HMO and threaten to leave the plan if they're ever kept waiting that long again. The HMO calls the clinic administrator and holds over his head the $20,000 a month that the HMO pays the clinic for covering their customers. The administrator then finds the root of the "problem," namely, the fresh-faced doctor who took time with his patients. The young doctor is told that if he doesn't see his patients on time, he's fired.

There probably isn't an official "ten minutes per visit" policy. The HMO would probably be shocked if it learned that a doctor was telling patients to shut up and not ask questions. But for the doctor on the front lines, trying to keep costs down for his clinic, and ultimately for the HMO, it's the only way to survive in the high-pressure managed care environment.

"I was so shocked that I didn't press him."

Patients have a long way to go before they get over that shock. Most of us still think of health care as a right, necessity, or gift. Most of us think of medicine in terms of the comforting face of Dr. Marcus Welby, and of course, HMOs try to give us this image in their ads. We desperately want to be put at ease, especially during an exam like Mara's. We still think that all we have to say is "Fix me up, doc," and all the resources of modern medical technology will be at our feet.

But health care is business. HMOs operate on tight margins and take huge risks. Like any other business, they will try to extract the most value from every interaction. But unlike other businesses, customer service does not seem to be a priority in managed care. If Mara had been served the wrong meal at a restaurant, for instance, she undoubtedly would have pressed the waiter for the right response. Why didn't she do that here? Because it was the last place she would have expected to find rudeness and impatience. Even though we distrust our HMOs, we still let our doctors treat us like children.

"I refused to go back to that first doctor."

In Mara's HMO, the next doctor she sees might not be as rude, but will be just as rushed. And if Mara silently skips from one doctor to the next, her file will tell some doctor down the line that she is a difficult patient. Her paper trail will tell the story of a patient who is hard to please. As unjust as this may sound, it's true that doctors think about these things when they review a patient's file. There's a way around this: work with the doctor you've got. In the next few chapters, we'll show you how to turn a harried doctor into a helpful doctor, preserving the relationship that forms the foundation of good treatment.

Instead of working past the rudeness we encounter in our health plans, most of us complain to our friends, stew silently, or vote with our feet. Others complain bitterly to administrators, countering rudeness with a belligerence that may never pierce these bureaucrats' thick hide. There might be a time when you have to deliver a failing report card about your doctor, but the first and best thing to do is to speak up and get his attention.

Back in the days when we saw doctors in private practice, there was, of course, no one to complain to but the doctor himself. Doctors knew this, and wouldn't dream of letting a patient walk away dissatisfied. But in managed care, many doctors know that you are stuck, and many know how few patients actually complain. This new system requires a new approach. We could dramatically improve our care if we chose to speak up.

"I found out she wasn't a doctor, but a nurse practitioner."

Under managed care, we see many fewer doctors than we used to. It's all part of cost-containment—nurse's salaries aren't as high as doctors', and as HMOs try to keep their profits up, nurse practitioners will be called upon more and more frequently to give advice, care, and prescriptions. If the nurse practitioner is properly trained and supervised, the system actually makes a lot of sense. And as we will see later, the savings are often passed on to the consumer.

But clearly, Mara was disappointed when she got to the office and found she wasn't going to see a doctor at all. The rule of thumb in dealing with HMOs is to assume nothing. If there's a way to cut costs, they will do it.

"So she pulled out a stack of cards from Planned Parenthood."

There are times when you should go outside of your HMO for a test or service. This isn't one of them. Confidentiality in this case is a smokescreen. Every patient the nurse practitioner sends to Planned Parenthood for a test saves her employer money. When the HMO reviews her cases, and sees how little her patients have cost them, she is rewarded with bonuses. From the standpoints of public and personal health, the NP has done exactly the wrong thing by discouraging someone who could be easily tested right then and there. The fact that she has a stack of cards ready suggests that she's done the very same thing many times before, which is unfortunate.

The result? Mara once again puts off being tested. At this point, she's also completely forgotten her question about irregular periods, and it's unlikely that she will be able to take off work again to deal with these concerns. On top of that, she feels neglected and angry, and probably won't be inclined to visit her HMO again unless she's actually sick. She's now just the kind of customer the HMO accountants want.

Where Do My Premiums Go?

If Mara never again shows her face in the clinic that treated her so poorly, that clinic will still be paid. Mara's employer will still pay her HMO about $100 per month to cover all her needs. If she doesn't have any needs, her HMO pockets that money or uses it to cover patients who require more intense care. Again, this is called "capitation," and is at the heart of why she was rushed through the system. Let's take a look at how that $100 is divided.

About 15 percent goes to administrative costs. Ten percent goes directly to profit, leaving about $75 per month. One-half of that $75 is put away in case Mara is ever hospitalized. The other half ($37 a month, or about $440 a year) goes to the group of doctors who are responsible for her care. Her $440 goes into a pool with the payments, sometimes more, sometimes less, of perhaps 10,000 other patients, and that money has to pay those doctors whether they are treating ten patients a day or twenty patients a day.

Many of the doctors getting Mara's $440 per year are in specialty clinics, like the women's clinic she visited. The clinic might get as little as $3 per month from Mara's original $100. So clearly, they need that $3 per month from as many patients as they can get in order to cover overhead, salaries, and equipment. The administrator who oversees this clinic watches costs very tightly, and if he does well, he gets a bonus every six months. He's also rewarded for keeping referrals down, and obviously has no incentive to experiment with new life-saving treatments or tests. We think that as managed care evolves, this system of bonuses will be removed, either voluntarily or through regulation. But even if that happens, one thing will stay the same: the need to keep a tight lid on costs.

There's nothing inherently wrong with keeping costs down. The old way of practicing medicine allowed costs to run away at twice the rate of inflation for decades. Most health care consumers didn't mind or even notice—as long as someone else was paying the bill. And the fawning attention of doctors was easy to get used to. So let's take look at what might have happened if Mara had visited a private practice doctor under the traditional fee-for-service system. As we will see, the older system has some serious drawbacks of its own.

What's Wrong with the Old-Fashioned Way?

Did you know that the practice of getting health insurance from your employer became widespread only because of a historical accident? Trade unions had been fighting for benefits since the nineteenth century, but in 1940, only 12 million Americans had health insurance through their jobs. It took a world war to get many employers to offer this expensive benefit.

During the Second World War, the government froze wages to keep inflation under control. Employers faced a labor shortage, but couldn't offer higher salaries to attract workers; the War Labor Board, however, permitted them to compete for employees with benefits packages. Before long, offering health insurance was standard. After the war, the now-established practice continued, and by 1950, 77 million workers had health insurance through their employers. No one planned this system, but it was very easy for us to get used to.

We got the best care money could buy when we were under traditional indemnity plans. We chose our doctors, paid our deductibles, and probably didn't even think about how much it cost beyond that. Doctors and hospitals knew this, and they did pretty well. The conventional treatment strategy called for tests to check every possibility, no matter how remote. Every advance in medical science was a new opportunity to increase costs. But the most important difference between the fee-for-service system and managed care is this: under a fee-for-service or indemnity plan, each patient who walked through a doctor's door was a benefit. Under managed care, each patient who asks for care is a cost.

So what would have happened if Mara had indemnity insurance? She walks into the office of Dr. Rich, a doctor she chose. This doctor takes her time. Mara first sees her in an opulent office, with pictures of the babies Dr. Rich has delivered and souvenirs from exotic vacation spots. The doctor has reviewed Mara's medical history, as well as her insurance plan. During their conversation, designed to gain Mara's trust, Dr. Rich learns that Mara is a doctor as well. They establish rapport, and then adjourn to the examining room.

Mara now asks about HIV screening. The doctor offers to do the test in-house, and give her the results that day. She then suggests a baseline mammogram, which can be done by her associates. In answer to Mara's irregular periods, she recommends that her hormone levels be checked with yet another test. She also tells Mara to monitor her periods closely and come back for a follow-up in a few months. In passing, Mara mentions a new blood test she's read about called CA-125. The test will tell Mara if she's in a high-risk group for ovarian cancer. Dr. Rich doesn't hesitate to add this to the battery of tests already planned.

Mara is what they call a "good" patient, meaning she has good insurance. She gets the maximum care the system can offer. The doctor extracts the maximum value from the visit. Mara leaves feeling listened to, respected, and well treated. So what's the problem? Let's take a closer look at Mara's visit with Dr. Rich.

That long conversation Mara had with Dr. Rich wasn't charity work. Dr. Rich is in demand, and will charge $300 for an initial consultation, $150 for each follow-up visit. So she has no need to see six patients an hour. She also knows that Mara's insurance plan will allow her to go down the road to Dr. Wealthy any time. In this situation, it pays to be polite.

Dr. Rich's offer to get results from the HIV screening the same day is welcome. It's hard to wait for days for a result as important as this. But if Mara had to pay herself, would she be so eager for the expedited test? The difference can be hundreds of dollars. Most people in this situation would put up with the wait, but Mara doesn't have to— her insurance company will handle it.

A hormone test *might* get to the root of Mara's irregular periods, but chances are the answer to the problem can be arrived at much more simply. Has Mara actually tracked her irregularities? How serious are they? Does she have a real reason to be concerned? Would an oral contraceptive prescription take care of the problem? These questions do not enter the doctor's mind—a test is the answer to everything.

And while we're on the subject of tests, why is Mara getting a CA-125? Does she have particular reason to think she is in a high-risk group? Does she realize that this test is still new and might give her an ambiguous result? Even worse, this and other tests carry the risk of "false positives," which would lead to even further tests, and possibly invasive procedures.

Every time we subject ourselves to a test or procedure, even a screening test, we put ourselves at risk. The problem is more widespread than you might think. One-fifth of all patients who leave a hospital take with them an infection or some other more serious problem that they didn't have when they checked in. An average of 180,000 patients die preventable deaths each year due to human error, mistaken judgment, or negligence. The sad thing is that so many of these tests, so many of these procedures that prove ultimately harmful, have been performed unnecessarily.

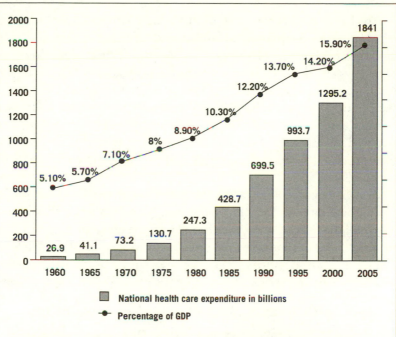

Figure 1.3. Past and Projected National Health Care Expenditures
Source: Health Care Financing Administration

With Medicare, Medicaid, and indemnity insurance picking up the tab, doctors and hospitals could spend freely. Even with managed care in place, health care will continue to take more of our nation's wealth as the baby boom bubble moves into their senior years.

A study by the Rand Corporation in 1988, when less than 40 million Americans were enrolled in HMOs, examined in detail a wide sampling of procedures and found that 25 percent of them were "questionable." Even the numbers for serious and invasive procedures were high. Looking at coronary angiographies (which diagnose blockages in heart arteries), the author of the study found that 17 percent were "inappropriate." Another 9 percent were "questionable."

Tests aren't the only things that have been overdone. The cesarean section is a frequently needed operation, but why was it on the rise? By the mid-eighties, 23 percent of our children were born by cesarean— 8 percent more than the rate recommended by the Department of Health and Human Services and twice the rate in Western European countries.

Are European women just stronger than American women? Or could it have something to do with the fact that hospitals can charge an extra $4,000 for each cesarean? How many of these and other procedures were done just because someone—namely, an insurer— would pay for it? How much suffering has medical science caused in the pursuit of higher billing? Even a relatively noninvasive and "low-risk" screening test such as a blood test for cancer can lead to a tremendous amount of mental anguish, especially if the result is a false positive (the term for a result that falsely indicates the patient has the disease).

Even if our hypothetical Dr. Rich did what she believed was in Mara's best interest, the practice of piling up bills has a social cost. When all the tests are done, and the follow-up visits complete, who pays for the $2,000 of tests that were ordered on Mara's behalf? We all do.

The insurance company raises its premiums, passing the cost of Mara's tests on to everyone covered by the plan. Mara's employer sees

---

WISHFUL THINKING ABOUT MEDICARE AND MEDICAID

When President Johnson signed Medicare and Medicaid into law in 1965, projections of how much it would cost were as optimistic as the era. The analysts said that by 1990, the costs of the program would be around 9 billion dollars. A bargain.

In 1990, we spent 70 billion dollars on these programs.

In 1993, the cost was up to 128.8 billion.

A MANAGED CARE TIMELINE

1910–1916 Doctors Thomas Curran and James Yocum transform their Western Clinic in Tacoma, Washington, into a pre-paid group plan. Local mill workers get coverage for fifty cents per month.

1927 The U.S. Congress forms the Committee on Costs of Medical Care to address "excessive" health care costs. Hospital stays then cost about four dollars a day.

1929 A group of fifteen hundred schoolteachers in Baylor, Texas, form a group plan that would later become Blue Cross Insurance Company. Six dollars a year covered an enrollee for twenty-one hospital days.

1935 National health insurance removed from the Social Security Act.

1938 Dr. Sidney Garfield contracts with Kaiser Corporation, then a construction company, to provide prepaid care to five thousand workers building the California Aqueduct.

1945–1950 Kaiser Corporation gives up on construction, and becomes a health care company. By the mid-sixties, Kaiser was insuring one million lives; today the company spends over $10 billion on health care every year.

1965 Medicare and Medicaid added to Social Security.

1960s Dr. Paul Ellwood develops the concept of a health care system centered on private health companies operating in open markets and watched over closely by government regulation. He coins the term "health maintenance organizations" to describe such companies.

1973 The Nixon administration–sponsored "HMO Act" becomes law. Government grants go out to qualified HMOs to help with start-up costs.

1983 The federal government tries to get a handle on Medicare and Medicaid costs by fixing prices for five hundred categories of diagnoses. Instead of controlling costs, diagnoses for more expensive medical problems rise by 10 to 13 percent.

1988 AlliedSignal, a Fortune 500 aerospace company, offers its eighty thousand employees coverage by an HMO for a lower payroll deduction. The company saves millions of dollars in health care costs.

1992 General Motors announces a $23.5 billion loss. The company places blame on its employee benefit and retirement packages, which GM says add $1,400 to the cost of each car. Expenditures for health insurance, claims GM, are higher than expenditures on steel.

1993 As health care premiums rise an average of 10 percent nationwide, the California Public Employees Retirement System gets a 0.7 percent reduction by negotiating with an HMO.

1993 President Clinton's Healthcare Security Act introduced. The reform fails due to insurance industry lobbying and public apathy.

1994 Thanks to mass migration to HMOs, average health benefits paid by employers decrease for the first time ever.

1996 Newborns' and Mothers' Health Protection Act signed into law, halting practice of "drive-through" deliveries.

1998 President Clinton's Patient Bill of Rights dies in Congress.

1999 Nationwide, 440,000 Medicare patients are dropped from HMOs. Average premiums for all patients go on the rise by 5 to 9 percent.

the premium increase, subtracting from the company's bottom line, so raises and bonuses are lower for everyone the following year. The government receives less in payroll taxes from Mara and her colleagues, less in taxes from the insurance company, and pays out more in Medicare and Medicaid costs to Dr. Rich and the many other doctors operating under the same assumptions. We all know what that means—higher taxes. We all pay for unnecessary tests and procedures.

What's wrong with old-fashioned health care is that no one has an interest in questioning, for example, whether Mara needs same-day HIV screening results. Those unnecessary costs paid for by indemnity insurance really add up. By 1994, we were spending 14 percent of our gross domestic product on health care. That's one out of every seven dollars spent in this country. Two billion dollars a day. Four thousand dollars per person per year. Real money.

But now the pendulum has swung to the other side. Instead of living in a free-spending health care system, we are at the mercy of penny-pinching managed care administrators. No one seems to be looking for a middle ground. Our employers are sick of paying high premiums, and managed care is the only relatively inexpensive option. So it falls to us—the actual patients in managed care—to work in, with, and sometimes against the system we've been dropped into.

How Can This Book Help?

When we looked around at how other books for patients grapple with the problem of managed care, we knew we had to offer a different approach. Too many of these guides advocate a "take on your doctor" approach. Patients were being told that they should question their doctor's every move, ask him how he is paid, and make sure an HMO bureaucrat isn't controlling him. We know that's the wrong way.

At the same time, many of these guides made patients think that they should expect the same care and attention that they got under the old system. We know that's wrong as well. For one thing, we aren't convinced the old system was that great, as we just discussed. For another thing, it's just not realistic. We can't go back.

When you read this book, you will get to see many ugly things about managed care. We are sorry to say that you will also get to see the ugly sides of a few of our physician colleagues. But just because we think you should work with them doesn't mean we think you should accept inferior care. The doctor who treated Mara was dead wrong to talk to her in the way that he did. When you are in a situation like that, you can either try to win the doctor over to your side or you can fume about how you have been mistreated. Only the first way will help get your medical problems resolved.

So please keep in mind that we are talking about the way things are, not the way we think things should be. When you left indemnity insurance and signed up for managed care, you traded your Lexus for a used Honda. You expect your Honda to work, but you don't expect it to have every frill your Lexus had. You will sometimes have to gently coax it up a hill. You will have to spend a little more time at the repair shop. Your managed care plan is the same way. It will get you where you want to go, but you have to put a little more work into it yourself.

The other thing we noticed about the current HMO self-help books is the fact that preventive medicine is left completely out of the picture. That's a real problem for us, since we know that a little pre-vention can help you avoid most of the problems associated with HMOs. In fact, HMOs should be working day and night on ways to get their patients into preventive programs. It's a common-sense way to produce real savings, but they just don't do it.

That's how this book was hatched. Dr. Theodosakis, director of the Preventive Medicine Residency Training Program at the University of Arizona College of Medicine, has seen how lives can change with a little preventive push. Dr. Feinberg, medical director for managed care and outpatient services at the UCLA Neuropsychiatric Institute and Hospital, has an insider's view of how managed care treats and mis-treats patients. When we talked about what this book should do, we realized that we couldn't just paint a rosy picture for you. The realities of managed care are tough. But we can give you the tools to pull you and your family through.

Each chapter addresses a specific part of managed care, and delivers immediately useful tips on how to improve your experience with your HMO. Our appendices cover issues related to specific diseases, and include forms to help you with your information. Here's a rough guide to what you will find in this book.

The next chapter you will read covers the reasons why you shouldn't let your relationship with your doctor go bad. Even if he's a pill, there are ways you can get through. There is a real person behind that brusque and hurried manner. You will need that person on your side.

Chapter 3 shows you how to make it through the ten-minute office visit. There's a simple method for delivering medical information. All doctors know it, and now that ten minutes is all you have, it's time to start speaking their language. The method you will learn is called HEAD.

Chapter 4 is a quick guide to problem doctors and how to get through to them using the method taught in chapter 3. We also show you how to tell if you have a real lemon on your hands, and when you should switch physicians.

Chapter 5 is devoted entirely to the high road to health—prevention. Here you will learn not just the basics, but also how to make your HMO a partner in prevention.

Chapter 6 covers what you will need to do if you get sick. Your HMO will often try to give you the cheapest treatment. This chapter will show you how to get the best.

Chapter 7 hits HMOs where they live. Denial of care is the single most frustrating and life-threatening thing that can happen to a patient. In this chapter, we show you how to appeal, and how to use the magic words "medically necessary."

Chapter 8 will help you watch out for your children in managed care. They have special needs, and are at special risk in an HMO. We'll show you how to keep those risks at a minimum.

Chapter 9 is for seniors, but anyone who has an elderly relative in managed care should read this short chapter as well. Everyone over sixty-five in managed care should have an advocate, and this advocate could be you.

Chapter 10 clears the muddied waters of psychiatric managed care. This is the care that health plans love to deny more than any other, but it's care that many of us really need. This behind-the-scenes look at what happens in the HMO's mental health wing will prepare you for the struggles of managed mental health care.

The final chapter provides a brief look at what might happen to managed care if the trends we see today continue. But since no one knows where it's really headed, we also use this chapter to share our dream of where we'd like it to go.

But you don't have to wait for that dream to be realized to make managed care work for you today. The realities of managed care are manageable. Anyone can do it. In the coming chapters, we will show you how.

RESOURCES FOR MORE INFORMATION ON OUR HEALTH CARE SYSTEM

Alliance for Health Reform
1900 L Street NW
Washington, DC 20036
(202) 466–5626
www.allhealth.org
Publishes briefs and position papers on managed care issues.

Employee Benefits Research Institute
2121 K Street NW
Washington, DC 20037
(202) 659–0607
www.ebri.org
Both corporations and unions support this organization, which publishes findings on all sorts of employee benefits and compensation arrangements.

Foundation for Accountability
520 SW 6th Street
Portland, OR 97204
(503) 223–2228
www.facct.org
Collects data on health plans, mostly for employers, but has many publications for consumers as well.

American Association of Health Plans
1129 20th Street NW
Washington, DC 20036
(202) 778–3200
www.aahp.org
The largest trade organization for HMOs, with 1,000 members.

Health Care Financing Administration
7500 Security Blvd.
Baltimore, MD 21244
www.hcfa.gov
The government agency that oversees Medicare and Medicaid programs. The website also provides general information on managed care issues.

~ 2 ~
Finding Compassion in the Managed Care Maze

QUESTIONS THIS CHAPTER ANSWERS

◆ Why is a good relationship with my doctor so important?

◆ What are the different types of plans, and how is my relationship with my doctor different in each?

◆ What is my doctor really thinking about?

◆ How has managed care changed my doctor's role?

◆ How can I form a trusting, mutual relationship with my doctor?

◆ How can I keep the HMO out of the examining room?

Sharon was happy with her doctor, happy with her care, and happy with her plan. What she wasn't happy with were the enormous premiums her indemnity insurance hit her with each month. It was time to shop around. Wading through the unfamiliar landscape of managed care, she came across a familiar face. Her physician, Dr. Yes, was on the list of a managed care plan that would cost her half as much as her indemnity plan. That made her choice very easy. "He was an older doctor," Sharon said, "and he would always spend time with me. I knew I could always reach him by phone if I had any questions. I chose my new insurance specifically because his name was on their list."

Sharon thought the change would be invisible. Same doctor, same patient, same health concerns, same treatment. Like so many of us who signed up for managed care, however, she soon realized that you just can't get the same service for half the cost. To Dr. Yes, the change was far from invisible. Sharon went from an insurance company that paid Dr. Yes in the neighborhood of $150 per visit, no questions asked, to an intrusive HMO that paid him perhaps $10 a month to cover all of Sharon's visits. To Sharon, it was a wise consumer choice. To Dr. Yes, it looked like a betrayal.

Sharon was amazed at how quickly Dr. Yes learned to say no: "He just stopped returning my calls, and I even had a hard time getting in to see him. When I finally talked to him, I was livid. I was a longtime patient, and I thought we had a good relationship. I knew he was completely changed because of the money and I told him so. I lost it. I yelled and he yelled back—and I'm never going to see him again."

Both doctor and patient in this case haven't accepted the realities of managed care. Dr. Yes hasn't come to terms with the fact that his fee-for-service patients can't keep up with their premiums. He hasn't learned to leave his concerns about money at the examining room door. Thanks to his HMO, he is seeing more patients, but getting less money per case. He hasn't found the time to return all their calls.

Sharon also has a lot to learn about managed care. She picked a bargain, and thought that she would get the same service for less money—an assumption she would probably never make about any other service business. If she were at her hairdresser's, would she have any reason to expect a shampoo, perm, and trim for the same price as a trim? Even if she has a great relationship with her stylist? Both patients and doctors are still learning to cope with health care as a business.

Communication between doctors and patients breaks down when money is in the middle. Patients have to realize that they won't get everything they used to get from doctors, and balance that against their needs. Taking that step means we have to show a bit more empathy with our doctors, but still know where to draw the line.

We tend to blame the doctor when things go wrong. He *should* be the one making the decisions, he's the one bringing us the bad news, and he's the one we've put our trust in (after all, who would trust an HMO?). When our doctor doesn't take time with us, when he doesn't seem compassionate enough, or when he says with a straight face, "Your plan won't pay for that," our faith in the doctor-patient relationship is shaken to the core. It is through a strong doctor-patient relationship, however, that healing starts. We can't let our HMOs come between us and our doctors.

This chapter will be devoted to how you can improve that relationship with your doctor. We're about to look behind the curtain to understand why our physicians are acting so strangely. What are they really thinking about as we explain our problems and concerns? What do they think of their bosses and medical directors at the HMO? What effect do their contracts with managed care organizations have on their professional judgment? How can we get our doctors to start acting like doctors again instead of insurance agents? The first step is to understand how our HMOs treat our doctors.

This chapter has two parts. First, we cover the different types of managed care organizations to help you understand the bureaucracy that surrounds your doctor. The second part is devoted to explaining why the cherished doctor-patient relationship has collapsed under the weight of the HMOs. Once you understand why, you will have the power to start rebuilding that relationship. In almost every case, you will find your doctor a willing partner.

Mutuality:
The New Model for Doctor-Patient Relationships

As we looked through recently published guides to dealing with your HMO, we found a disturbing trend. Various popular strategies for making your way through the managed care maze too often advocate an adversarial approach to talking with your doctor. They too seldom offer insight into what she must deal with on a minute-by-minute basis. Each patient who comes to the doctor produces a snarl of paperwork and regulations, oversight and reviews, and legal and ethical problems. And then the patient has to be cured. If all patients follow the advice of the "take on your doctor" approach, they create just one more headache for a skilled professional who already has too much on her mind.

But the old doctor-patient relationship, where the doctor made all the decisions and only gave the patient information on a "need to know" basis, won't work either. Today's health care consumers are informed and demanding. They have been trained to question—and they should question. The trick is to question in a way that doesn't build walls between you and your doctor.

In their study of the doctor-patient relationship, Debra L. Roter and Judith A. Hall found four types of relationships. Doctor control and patient control define the relationships. The very best relation-

The Four Types of Doctor-Patient Relationships

Doctor control

		Low	High
Patient control	**Low**	*Default* Both patient and doctor unhelp-ful. Lack of mutual respect and trust. Problem not defined, solution not found.	*Paternalistic* Doctor doesn't trust patient. Doctor thinks he knows best. Doctor left to find decision on his own. Patient intimidated by doctor. Patient doesn't question doctor's treatment plan.
	High	*Consumerism* Patient doesn't trust doctor. Patient questions every decision. Patient doesn't follow treatment plan. Doctor hemmed in by patient on one side, HMO on the other.	*Mutuality* Mutual respect and trust. Doctor and patient team up to find a solution. Doctor listens to patient's needs. Patient follows treatment plan he helped create.

Adapted from Debra L. Roter and Judith A. Hall, *Doctors Talking with Patients/Patients Talking with Doctors* (Westport, CT: Auburn House, 1992).

ship occurs when both doctor and patient know they have control. The four types of relationships are default, consumerism, paternalism, and mutuality. We believe you should always try for a mutual relationship with your doctor.

Since HMOs are big business, it's always tempting to act like a consumer in the examining room. But that takes away your doctor's power to heal you. On the other hand, it's always tempting for doctors to act like they know best, to have a parental-type relationship with their patients. But in the space of a ten-minute office visit, all you are likely to get is the stern parent, rather than the caring one.

We have to learn how to ask our questions without aggravating our doctors. We have to take control of the visit without taking away the doctor's power to heal. We have to show him that he can't treat us like children, but at the same time give him the respect he deserves.

The very best way to creating a mutual relationship is to learn how your doctor thinks. Take into account how he is pressured by the HMO, how he is being asked to save money by denying care, and how he is paid. Then, after you have considered his position, get him on your side. Once he is on your side, he will be ready to join you in the fight to get the best, and not just the cheapest, medical care.

HMO, IPA, PPO, POS:
What Do They Mean to Me and My Doctor?

Managed care is an evolving system. Plans are being rapidly developed, tested, and then dropped just as quickly as they came up. Companies are integrating services, spinning off services, upsizing, and downsizing in a "Goldilocks syndrome" as they look for the mixture that's just right. To consumers, the result looks more like Frankenstein's monster than an orderly experiment, but either way, we are the subjects. It might surprise you to learn that your doctor is also being experimented with. In many ways, he's even more closely watched, more deeply probed, and viewed with even more suspicion than you are. For a number of reasons, he often has even less opportunity to take control of this nationwide trial in managed care.

In all of the types of arrangements we are about to discuss, control is exercised over doctors in similar ways. First, and this is a key to managed care, you usually need to see a primary care physician (PCP) before you see a specialist. This is generally called "gatekeeping." Everyone does it. Gatekeeping results in savings when the less-expensive PCP treats a minor problem on his own, rather than sending you to a more expensive specialist. The basic idea is to have someone grant "permission" before you start using the HMO's more expensive services.

Each type of plan has its own system for referrals in place. Some plans allow PCPs to refer only to specialists in the same building; some allow them to refer to specialists in a looser "network." Some plans allow you to refer yourself, but only with a higher co-payment. We will discuss these differences in turn.

The other element all managed care organizations share is "utilization review." This is a review of patients' use of services. Sometimes it involves a single case, sometimes it involves looking at how much all the patients in a plan use a particular service. The review is usually performed by utilization review (UR) doctors and nurses. The UR doctors never meet patients, but their decisions can override the decisions of the PCP, and have a direct impact on treatment options. We will be discussing the UR doctor's role later in this book.

It would be dull and pointless to take you through each current and possible plan—many of them won't be around by the time you read this. Instead, we will focus on the three major types of plans—HMO, POS, and PPO. Each one presents challenges to a successful relationship with your doctor. Each one offers the doctor challenges that seem to be his alone, but which you can help him resolve.

The HMO: Vanilla-Flavored Managed Care

This is the plan most of us think of when we think of managed care, but as the experiment progresses, this "traditional" managed care plan accounts for less market share, inspiring little confidence that it will be the plan of the future. Of the three plans we will discuss—health maintenance organization (HMO), point-of-service option (POS), and preferred provider organization (PPO)—the HMO offers the least choice, the fewest options, and the tightest control.

But there's a trade-off: the HMO is generally the lowest-priced of the managed care plans. Employers who offer a range of plans typically offer the HMO option with little or no paycheck deduction. Only a small number of HMOs (around 20 percent) have a deductible, usually about $200.

The HMO is the most basic form of managed care, though it still comes in a variety of packages—staff model, group model, independent practice association (IPA) model, and mixed model. The differences may not be apparent to the patient in the waiting room, but they can make all the difference to your doctor. So to help you understand him, we should take a little time with each one before exploring the PPO and POS options.

We should point out that these are *models*, and that particulars about the plan may vary from company to company. But the important thing to understand is where your doctor fits into his organization. Once you find out how your doctor is being treated, you can develop a strategy for getting the best treatment from your doctor.

The Staff Model HMO

If your health plan sends you to what looks like a hospital, you are probably with a staff model HMO. The organization typically owns

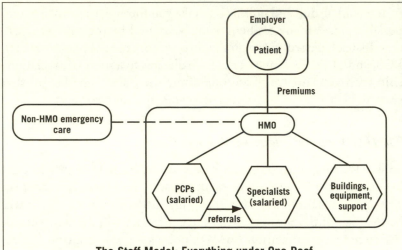

The Staff Model: Everything under One Roof

In a staff model, the patient and the patient's employer's premiums go to support not just the doctors, but the infrastructure of the hospital-like care center. In the event of an emergency, patients may use non-HMO care, but otherwise, they are limited to the services contained in the HMO. Primary care physicians may only refer patients to specialists who are part of the same HMO.

the buildings, equipment, and offices, which is why start-up costs for this type of venture are so high. The idea, often referred to as "vertical integration," is to offer one-stop shopping for health care needs, even going beyond the goals of the conventional hospital. Having everything in one place can be great for elderly or chronically ill patients. They don't have to run all over town to see different specialists and fill prescriptions. All they need is in one building.

But the convenience of having everything in one place also limits choice. Members of a staff model HMO cannot seek unapproved nonemergency care outside the HMO. Even emergency care given outside the HMO is frequently questioned after the fact, adding financial trauma to an already traumatic situation. Patients in a staff model often feel shuffled around and tightly controlled. They need a referral from their primary care physician for just about any problem. And since they often don't know who they will see when they come in for an appointment, they have a more difficult time forming relationships with their doctors.

Doctors in this system are just as bound by the cost-cutting rules and dictates as the patient. Most of them are on the clock. They might get bonuses, stock options, or profit-sharing in addition to a salary, but their salaries are the baseline. They are always much less than the salaries of the HMO executives.

We can't overemphasize how different this is from the old system. Doctors used to have more in common with the entrepreneur than the company man. They set their own rates, hours, vacation times, and retirement. Giving a doctor a salary, even when it's much higher than what most of us get, is like putting a cat on a leash. Doctors have been trained to question, analyze, and figure out problems for themselves. The majority of them still remember the days when a comfortable private practice was their reward for years of medical school tuition payments and sleepless residencies.

There's a good chance that your doctor is still wondering how he wound up in managed care. If you want him to pay attention to your needs, you don't want to remind him, even in a subtle way, that he's working for an HMO.

The Group Model HMO

The group model is slightly more complex and designed to get around the staff model's high start-up costs. In this arrangement, the HMO negotiates contracts with medical groups—clinics, multi-doctor practices, single-specialty groups, or multi-specialty practices—which in turn hire and manage doctors. The HMO does not own the medical group, but in most cases, the medical group has an exclusive relationship with the HMO. That means that doctors in the group can only see patients covered by the HMO. The group practice is effectively an extra layer between the physician and the HMO, and can be more flexible in attracting doctors with different compensation packages.

Some doctors may be on salary, just as they are in a staff model. Some may be compensated on a "cost" basis—they are paid a set amount for seeing patients, and a set amount for performing procedures preapproved by the plan. Or they might get paid based on how many patients are on the HMO's roster. Some group models even offer doctors profit-sharing arrangements in addition to salary or cost,

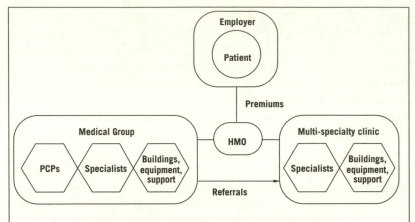

The Group Model: Managed Care under Many Roofs

In a group model, the HMO does not own the buildings and equipment, but serves as administrator for several coordinated medical groups, clinics, and hospitals. These institutions have long-term contracts with the HMO, and agree to see only patients from that HMO. Patients will usually go to a PCP in one medical group, who can refer them to specialists in their own group or to specialists in another clinic or hospital that's part of the same HMO.

with doctors fully sharing the risk. But any way the pie is sliced, the HMO is looking for one thing: financial incentives to doctors for keeping costs down.

Mara's OB-GYN, whom we introduced in the previous chapter, is cooperating fully with his organization by trying to see as many patients as possible and limiting their visits to ten minutes. He plays the game, and loses some of his freedom to make medical decisions in the process. If the HMO does well, he will get a bonus at the end of the year. Even though doctors participating in a group model are on a slightly longer leash than their colleagues in a staff model, many of them realize that working for a group rather than being on staff provides only an illusion of independence.

Patients in a group model need to be more active than patients in a staff model. Doctors in different groups work in different ways, even if they are part of the same HMO. Paperwork moves slowly between the various groups and the central HMO. Patients get frustrated when one doctor doesn't know what happened just last week in another location. After all, they assume, it's on the chart. Why shouldn't he know?

When patients take this frustration out on doctors, they lose their most valuable allies. When patients helpfully give updates on their treatments, or even bring a copy of their medical records, they gain the respect and gratitude of their doctors. Believe us, in these complicated organizations, you need all the friends you can get.

Group models and staff models were predominant during the early days of managed care, but are now in steady decline. In 1996, only about 10 percent of all HMOs were group or staff models, and their numbers have continued to decline as consumers demand more choice and flexibility from their health plans. One way HMOs have tried to deliver is with the independent practice association (IPA) model.

The IPA (Independent Practice Association) Model HMO

The IPA model is an attempt to find middle ground between the group model and the traditional indemnity plan. Under indemnity insurance, you faced no restriction on your choice of physicians. An HMO can't give you that, but it can broaden the range of your available choices.

As it turns out, the best way to offer more choice to consumers is to offer more choice and fewer restrictions to physicians. The IPA model follows the group model with one major difference: physicians are allowed to maintain their private practices. They are not obliged to make exclusive arrangements with an HMO. They can see patients from another HMO, or they can see patients who pay top dollar for indemnity insurance. The IPA acts very much like the medical group in the group model, but doesn't completely take away the doctor's independence.

This simple, subtle difference accounts for the IPA model's popularity. Patients are willing to pay a bit more just to be able to visit a doctor who is still in private practice. Over 44 percent of patients in managed care are willing to dig a little deeper for improved choice and the comfort of seeing a doctor who *acts* the way doctors used to and has his own practice. But there's nothing old-fashioned about the way he is paid.

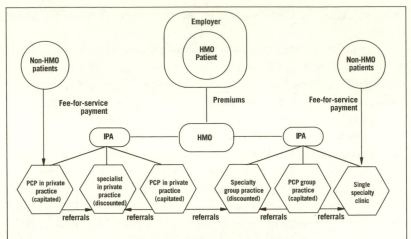

The IPA Model: A Managed Care Village

In an IPA model, the providers aren't contained by an HMO's or medical group's organization. Instead they sign individual contracts with the IPA, which acts as broker for the HMO. The individual doctors can sign additional contracts with other IPAs or HMOs. They can also see non-HMO patients, receiving a fee-for-service payment. This helps them minimize the risk of taking on HMO patients for a flat rate.

The HMO sends money to the IPA, which then pays the primary care physician a fixed per-patient fee based on how many enrollees choose him off the list. Again, this practice of prepaying a per capita rate is called "capitation." So far, it's very much like the group model, and nothing like the fee-for-service or indemnity model.

How does this give the patient greater choice? For one thing, the primary care physician (PCP) is also taking patients who will pay even more for fee-for-service treatment. He can even make up what he's losing from HMO patients by "cost shifting," that is, by charging more to fee-for-service patients. So more doctors will join the IPA because they don't have to give up their private practice.

Choice also comes to the IPA model through a different fee structure for specialists. They get a "discounted fee-for-service" payment, which amounts to another compromise. Banking on the idea that the IPA will keep their schedules full, they accept a lower payment for the HMO patients who walk through their doors. This is not capitation— if no patients come, no money is paid—but it has the same effect.

Their practices have to become volume businesses to survive. They can only offer a discount because the HMO keeps their waiting rooms full.

To many, the IPA model seemed like the answer to our problems. But it is an answer that poses many questions. Is the PCP giving equal care to every patient, or is he taking extra time with his fee-for-service patients and rushing his HMO patients out the door? Are doctors in a single IPA forced to compete with each other for patients? Will they make promises they can't keep? Medical ethics has only begun to address these questions.

Unfortunately, the HMOs figured out something important long before both patients and doctors did: whoever controls the patients has the power. The only reason IPAs exist is that doctors fear their flow of patients will be cut off if they do not participate. The management structure and costs of an IPA just removes health care dollars from the doctors and ultimately health care from the patients.

But the advantage for patients is that they can see a doctor they choose on a regular basis. They have a good chance to build strong relationships with doctors, even if they're rushed, underpaid, or just fed up with managed care. However, as we observed in Sharon's story, even the best relationship with an IPA doctor won't be the same as the relationships we used to have with fee-for-service doctors. The relationship now requires a little more work, and a little more patience, from both the patient and the doctor.

The Mixed Model HMO

Sometimes the experiments with staff, group, and IPA model HMOs all come together in one plan. The mixed model, also called the "network model," HMO offers doctors the widest range of options. They can join as staff, through a group, or through an IPA. A mixed model HMO will also contract with hospitals.

These HMOs attempt to minimize risk by attracting a wide range of providers. Say your primary care doctor, who belongs to the mixed model HMO through his IPA, wants to refer you to a dermatologist to look at a rash. If he were with a simple IPA model HMO, he would only have the option of sending you to a dermatologist who is compensated with a discount fee-for-service arrangement. That's an

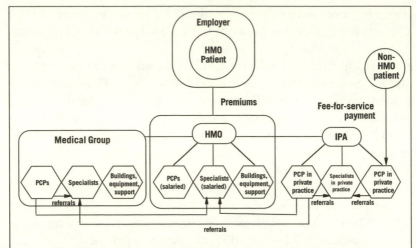

The Mixed or Network Model HMO: A Managed Care Metropolis

A mixed model HMO borrows all the ideas of the staff model, the group model, and the IPA model, and puts them all into practice at the same time. This allows them to be flexible in attracting doctors to the plan, and allows them to offer a wide range of options to the patients. On the downside, it's a very complex system, almost impossible for patients to figure out on their own. Even the doctors in the plan might not know the full reach of their HMO.

expensive option, and might make him rethink the referral. But if he's in a mixed model HMO, he can refer you to a skin care clinic that's part of the network. The clinic contracts with the HMO on the group model. That means it's fully capitated. They've already been paid to look at your rash. So your PCP isn't at risk for the referral. That makes it easier for you to get referrals.

It doesn't get much more complicated than this. Patients in the mixed model have the least idea of what's going on around them. Their doctors might be capitated, they might be getting a discounted payment, they might be on staff, or they might be seeing patients outside of the network. Who knows? How can you ever find out? Your doctor is the wrong person to ask. Money must be left out of the all-important doctor-patient relationship. But when you start wondering why it's easy to get a referral to a dermatologist and harder to get a referral to an ophthalmologist, it could be that they have very different financial relationships with your HMO.

We have just covered the HMO basics—staff model, group model, IPA model, mixed model—to help you not only identify your plan, but understand what your doctor is thinking about as he considers your treatment. All of these models are forcing your doctor to think about his place in the corporate food chain and breadline. In many ways, he can't help it. But you can help him clear his mind so he can be a doctor again. The first step is to understand what he is going through. The next step is to be an active, informed, and helpful patient. We'll get to that next step soon, but we still have to cover two additional types of health plans.

The POS Option: Managed Care with Something on the Side

The models we have discussed so far have one thing in common: patients cannot leave the network for nonemergency care without losing all coverage. When a groundswell of consumer complaints reached the HMOs' corporate offices, they realized that they had to offer a choice. The point of service option (POS) attempts to deliver. Here, patients can leave the HMO provider network for a price. Leaving the network means you give up the 100 percent coverage of the HMO for, typically, 70 percent coverage with a $250 deductible. Most non-network doctors are compensated the old-fashioned way: fee for service. So exercising the POS option is like turning back the clock to the days of indemnity.

The POS option is a relatively new idea, but one that caught on quickly. By 1992, about half of all HMOs offered the option. Three years later, almost three-quarters of our HMOs had adopted it. So far, it seems to be working for both consumers and organizations. Consumers like having the security of being able to see any doctor they want if the need arises. HMOs are at financial risk every time a patient goes outside of the network, but so far very few do. One survey by the American Association of Health Plans found that in half of the plans surveyed, only 10 percent of patients actually used their POS option. In most cases, it seems, the option of leaving the network is no more than a safety net.

Your PCP may not know if you have a POS option. He may not be allowed to encourage you to leave the network for a particular complaint. But there's nothing he can do to stop you, and as long as there isn't a paper trail to his examining room or practice, he won't be blamed for the increased cost to the organization when you exercise your option. He might even be relieved to know that you plan to leave the network for a certain complaint. There's a time and place to bring this up with your PCP, and it's usually after he's done all he can to help you. We'll discuss this in more detail in the next few chapters.

The PPO: A Managed Care Buffet

The preferred provider organization (PPO) was originally seen by many as a way to transition patients from an indemnity plan to an HMO. As it turns out, PPOs have offered serious competition to HMO plans and it seems like they are here to stay. Since 1993, enrollment in PPOs has grown at twice the rate of HMO enrollment, and PPOs now cover more lives than all HMOs combined. The IPA model is one way the HMOs are fighting back, and we may someday be unable to tell the difference between the HMO and the PPO without looking closely.

Here again, choice has its price. Employees who go the PPO route may see an extra 20 dollars a month deducted from their paychecks and pay deductibles of around $200. In return, they get to choose providers from a long list and have the option of leaving the network for a higher co-payment, just like the POS option.

But there is one very important difference. If you are with an HMO, most of your doctors are capitated. They get a flat rate for covering all your visits, no matter how many or how few. If you are with a PPO, most of your doctors get a discounted fee-for-service. They get paid only when you show up, and they agree to a smaller fee in exchange for increased patient volume, fewer delinquent bills, and faster bill payment. That's why PPOs are usually more expensive than HMOs.

Many PPOs allow patients to see an in-network specialist without a referral from a primary care physician. Those that don't allow this self-referral are called "gatekeeper model" PPOs, and are a slightly cheaper option. Either way, you are tied to the network. If you leave the network, you pay more and may have to pay out of pocket.

PPOs generally have a better reputation than the HMOs, but the buyer still has every reason to beware. Remember that discounted fee-for-service turns practices into volume businesses. The time pressure is still on—the ten-minute office visit can be found in the PPO as well as the HMO. There's also a big question about how far discounted fee-for-service really controls costs. If it fails, PPOs have few options: increase their patient base, cut their doctors' pay, or ask for higher premiums. Most likely, they will do all three. None of these strategies will make doctors or patients happy. All of them will put further strain on the doctor-patient relationship.

Now that we've placed the doctor in the system, we should take a closer look at how he is controlled by the system. This is just the next step toward understanding your doctor. By now it might not surprise

Managed Care at a Glance

	Staff HMO	Group HMO	IPA HMO	Mixed HMO	HMO with POS option	PPO
What's the monthly premium?	Single: $140 Family: $390	Single: $140 Family: $390	Single: $145 Family: $395	Single: $135 Family: $385	Single: $160 Family: $455	Single: $160 Family: $455
How much choice of doctors do I have?	None. Patients must see doctors on staff.	Limited. Patients see doctors in group practice.	Moderate. Patients may choose from a list of doctors in IPAs.	Moderate. Patients may get a choice, or may be sent to a medical group.	High. Patients may see non-network doctors for a 20% copayment	High. Patients may see network specialists without a referral.
How are doctors paid?	Salary.	Varies from group to group.	PCPs capitated, specialists get discounted fee-for-service.	Varies: Salary, capitated, or discounted fee-for-service.	Non-HMO doctors get fee-for-service when you exercise your option.	Discounted fee-for-service.
How much control does the plan exercise over doctors?	High. HMO administers doctors directly.	High. Group administers doctors.	Medium. Doctors allowed to see non-HMO patients.	Medium to high.	None for non-network doctors. Medium to high for network doctors.	Low. Many doctors face peer review rather than strict utilization review.
Where can my PCP refer me?	Only to other staff doctors.	To group doctors or doctors in other network groups.	To network doctors only.	To groups, network specialists, or staff.	Self-referrals okay with co-payment.	Patient can often self-refer, skipping over PCP "gatekeeper."

Note: The costs given are total monthly premiums. Some employers pick up the entire premium, some only pick up a percentage. The premiums given are national averages and are for comparison only. Actual costs vary widely from region to region, and are on the rise as this book goes to press.

you that she's not happy with managed care. But it may still surprise you how much she needs your help to avoid falling into the cost-control pitfalls that challenge her very identity as a doctor.

What Is My Doctor Really Thinking About?

It used to be so simple: doctor sees patient, takes tests, decides on treatment, follows up. Costs? What costs? Nothing more than "usual, reasonable, and customary," and nothing the insurance company won't handle. Now, at each stage, there's something else involved. Every decision must be checked against the balance sheet. Medicine wasn't supposed to be about money. Doctors' groups like the AMA put every effort into keeping commerce away from medicine. Now even the AMA knows that the capitalists are inside the gates. But for your doctor, this is about more than money. It's about the power to make decisions and help patients.

When that power is taken away, medical ethics are thrown off balance. A researcher at Tufts University claims that 70 percent of the doctors he talked to in an informal survey admitted to exaggerating or even lying about patients' symptoms for the patient's benefit. A patient with a headache, for example, might not get an MRI unless the doctor says he has blurred vision. A patient with hip pain might get ibuprofen instead of a more powerful drug unless the doctor claims he has an intolerance to the cheaper alternative. And a depressed patient might not get appropriate psychiatric care unless the doctor claims he has suicidal tendencies. It's disturbing to think about patients' medical records being falsified, but even more disturbing to think that these doctors feel compelled to commit fraud and violate their oaths in order to shepherd patients through the system.

There are just a few examples of the ethical problems posed by the new system of health care. In fact, there is no aspect to being a doctor that managed care has left untouched, and doctors don't like it. Polls of doctors regularly find that 30 to 50 percent of them wouldn't go to medical school if they had to decide all over again. In the first six months of 1994, as managed care malaise hit a peak, disability claims by doctors rose 60 percent.

Doctors looked at the care they provided, and they weren't happy with what they saw. In a 1997 study of California primary care physicians, a bare majority was "very" or "somewhat satisfied" with their ability to treat capitated patients according to their own best judgment, compared to 79 percent who were satisfied with their practice as a whole. When the doctors in the study were asked to rate their relationships with managed care patients, the response was similar. We can't have doctors who are unhappy with their work examining us.

The headaches doctors face today only increase outside the examining room. Managed care was supposed to cut down on paperwork, give doctors a cushion against malpractice suits, and provide job security with a steady stream of patients. It has done none of these things. Paperwork has only increased, and few HMOs take into account how time-consuming it can be. The system of bonuses for doctors who keep costs down makes for compelling arguments before juries. On the other hand, if costs aren't kept down, many physicians face the prospect of being "deselected."

"Deselection" or "delisting" is HMO-speak for getting fired. In most HMO contracts with physicians, this can happen for any reason, at any time. The law is currently trying to define doctors' rights in this area, but has a long way to go before doctors can rest easy. An HMO might terminate a doctor for overutilizing services, advocating too strongly for patients, pursuing back payments too forcefully, or criticizing the plan in front of patients. Patients may want to consider this last item during visits. You doctor may be sympathetic when you start complaining about the HMO, but he might be required by his contract to avoid joining you. One of these gag clauses was reported on by *Business Week* in 1996; the HMO responsible faced such a public uproar that it pulled the clause from its contracts in a matter of days. We can take a heartening lesson from this: health care consumers can put power back in the hands of doctors, even in cases where the doctors themselves can do nothing.

How Has Managed Care Changed My Doctor's Role?

Doctors have less control over their own lives than they used to. We can see this most clearly in the decline of private practice. From 1987 to 1997, the percentage of physicians in private practice dropped from 41 percent to 29 percent. Now, over 80 percent of primary care physicians have at least one managed care contract. Forty-five percent are employees of managed care organizations. We've mentioned how much professional power the doctor loses just by being inside an HMO's walls, but it goes even further than that. Managed care is eroding many of his functions, and much of his power, in the name of keeping costs down.

Gatekeeping is a much-abused term, but it describes a position of great decision-making power. In the medical pecking order, generalists or primary care physicians were often at the bottom, with specialists getting the research grants, the big salaries, and the journal bylines. Now the gatekeeper is much more than the first stop. He is the coordinator and manager of your health care. But even as the PCP assumed this new position of power, HMOs were taking it away. So-called "midlevel professionals," such as nurse practitioners and physician assistants, are being trained to keep the gates and even interpret lab work. Nurse practitioners are, in many locations, admitting patients into hospitals. You might never know this is happening when you get your lab work or are granted a hospital stay, but your doctor knows. The message he gets is that his once-central role is being challenged from all quarters.

The American Nursing Association has claimed that "60 to 80 percent of primary and preventative care, traditionally done by doctors, can be done by a nurse for far less money." While this might not automatically translate into 60 to 80 percent fewer PCPs, it does mean there will be fewer jobs. The job situation is already bad. We have around 17,000 medical students, and about 6,000 foreign-trained students, entering clinical training each year. By the year 2000, we are looking at 225 to 261 doctors per 100,000 consumers. HMOs typically hire based on the idea that around 100 doctors per 100,000 patients is "just right." HMOs that staff at 140 doctors per 100,000 patients are known as "physician favorable." It's an employers' market, and as medical school applications continue to rise, it will only get worse for doctors.

Your doctor performs a constant juggling act to keep her job. On the one hand, she's trying to control costs. On the other, she's trying to control quality. An enormous oversight mechanism monitors her every move. If she doesn't hit the exactly right balance between quality and economical care, she could be delisted.

Independence, decision-making, and job security are—and always have been—what give doctors the power and confidence they need to do their duty. That power has been weakened by managed care, but it isn't completely gone. When we put trust in our doctors and give them a problem to solve, we are putting power back in their hands. When we enter the waiting room ready to make the doctor an ally, in almost every case we will find him willing.

We aren't telling you all this just so you will feel sorry for our colleagues. We aren't just asking you to make their jobs easier. We are trying to help you understand that the current system drags doctors down. A doctor who has been laid low by managed care is useless to you. You want a doctor who is excited about his job, who likes patients, and who likes solving medical problems. With that motivating passion rekindled, you can begin building a mutual relationship that will set the stage for getting the best treatment.

We know that there is an inspired and compassionate doctor inside even the most downtrodden managed care burnout. We would like to show you how to bring that doctor out. When you do, the troubles of the HMO will disappear from the examining room. The money issues will vanish. All that will be left is a patient who needs help and a doctor who is ready to give it.

Why Did They Go to Medical School?

It's great being a doctor. We love our jobs, even in spite of all the challenges managed care has thrown in our career paths. Why? That's hard to put into words. Even Dr. William Carlos Williams couldn't put it into words, and he was one of America's greatest poets. As he wrote in his autobiography:

> We catch a glimpse of something, from time to time, which shows us that a presence has just passed us, some rare thing. . . . For a moment we are dazzled. What was that? We can't name it; we know it never gets into any reasonable avenue of expression. . . . Whole lives are spent in the tremendous affairs of daily events without even approaching the great sights I see every day.

We deal with the sick, we handle their bodily fluids, explore their cavities, and then we fill out insurance forms. Why would anyone want this job? Because we can, even if only now and then, catch that glimpse of "some rare thing." Like we said, it's hard to explain. The simple explanation is that we like patients.

Dr. Feinberg had such an experience in pediatrics when his hospital charged him with taking care of the tiniest baby ever born there. She was full-term, not premature, but had shared the womb with two others, and was almost vanishingly small. She received blood transfusions in exact amounts of less than half a teaspoon. Giving her even a drop more fluid than the precise dosage could have sent her into heart failure. Only Dr. Feinberg and one other colleague were allowed to perform this transfusion procedure on this particular patient. The hospital had to provide special calculators to figure her blood requirements because the standard ones couldn't carry the decimal points far enough.

Three months later, the baby was stable, but still in the hospital. Then one day, Dr. Feinberg was explaining her condition to her mother when she interrupted him for a question: "Can I hold her?" She had never held her baby. She had never asked. Dr. Feinberg and others had held the tiny infant, but no one had realized, in the middle of crunching those miniscule numbers, that the mother hadn't picked up her child. Dr. Feinberg said that of course she could, but as soon as he gave his nod of approval, she bolted out of the room.

Hours later she was back. Of course Dr. Feinberg had to ask why she had left. "I wasn't going to hold her in what I was wearing. I had to go home and shower and be in really nice clothes before I picked her up," she answered. In a strange way, that made the moment complete.

Almost every doctor has a story like this, and the stories almost always have two things in common that tell us why our doctors went to medical school. First, you have the science. Solving problems gets doctors' hearts pumping. How do you keep this tiny baby alive? What are her special needs and how does she change the routine procedures we take for granted? When we figure these things out, and see the results, it's a moment of perfection, a slam dunk. Give a doctor a problem to solve, and you will have his full attention.

But the picture isn't complete without the patient. In the middle of Dr. Feinberg's sixteen-hour days, lost in the science of counting drops of blood, the mother let him know what it all meant. Sometimes you just get lucky and get to see people in their lives, in parts of their lives that are—there's no other word for it—beautiful. HMOs make a considerable effort to make sure that their reviewers never see the patient. If they did, many more claims and requests would be approved. Give your doctor a beautiful life moment, and you will have his full attention, not just once, but for every visit and problem from that moment on.

How Can I Form a Trusting Relationship with My Doctor?

Doctors live for these cases that allow them to see people's lives in full. It might just be a glimpse, but we need to see these life-changing moments. Managed care has made that more difficult both for patients and doctors. Patients are becoming used to questioning everything the doctor does. They should question, but the questions should lead to trust.

Dr. Theodosakis has chosen to avoid working in a managed care environment. In fact, he jokes that he's one of the most privileged doctors in the country. His patients are mostly self-referred, well educated about their condition, and motivated to work with him as an active team member. Spared from wasting energy on daily battles with HMOs, Dr. Theodosakis has been free to focus on developing innovative treatment methods such as his program for arthritis, which is rapidly becoming the first-line therapy in the United States and several other countries.

Despite being able to practice in this way, Dr. Theodosakis still experiences the erosion of patient-medical system trust that has resulted from managed care. One patient who came to him had a particularly rare kind of heart disease that no one could treat. He had built a set of expectations about what the medical establishment could do for him, and felt that managed care had let him down. In truth, there just was no cure for his condition. When managed care didn't deliver, the patient built up a resentment toward all doctors, whether they were in managed care or not. There was no way Dr. Theodosakis could build trust with science in this case. The scientific cure wasn't there.

Luckily, Dr. Theodosakis knew that there are other ways to build a doctor-patient relationship. In cases like these, the doctor has to become a sort of spiritual counselor, teaching the patient to look at his condition from a different perspective. This particular patient had to learn to put his trust in his doctor rather than in science, and even further, had to learn to put his trust in himself. The treatment regimen prescribed by Dr. Theodosakis required the patient to completely change his outlook on life. He had to learn to accept that he would never be cured, even though he could maintain and live with his condition. Once he made this psychological leap, he wrote Dr. Theodosakis to let him know that his whole life had changed. Such feedback can be very important; in this case, it helped encourage Dr. Theodosakis to expand the patient's intervention.

Doctors are always eager to see the results of their work, and nothing gets to us quite like seeing the entire trajectory of a life change course. For the past nine years, Dr. Feinberg has been getting letters and pictures of a young girl he treated. This case—like that of the tiny baby—posed unusual challenges: the child inherited an enzyme deficiency that had only been recorded a few times before. The same condition had killed the mother's first child, so this time the condition was detected prepartum and the hospital was ready with a special formula that would replace the missing enzyme. The formula, unfortunately, would cause the baby to give off an extremely unpleasant and powerful odor. There were other problems. The mother was prone to depression and had been suicidal when her first baby didn't make it. Since Dr. Feinberg was headed for psychiatry, he was given the case.

Dr. Feinberg was in for the ride of his life. Before the baby was born, he set up the ICU to handle this special case, and when the baby was born he didn't leave her side. After overseeing all the preparation, there was no way he was going to relinquish control to someone else. The fact that he wasn't supposed to be working on the baby's first night didn't enter his mind. The fact that the formula the baby had to take produced such an offensive side effect didn't enter his mind. Here again, the chance to solve a problem made everything else trivial.

The baby did well, but the mother didn't. Her postpartum depression made her suicidal. Then she admitted that she wanted to kill the baby. Now it was a postpartum psychosis. The mother's regular therapist was on vacation, so Dr. Feinberg became her psychiatrist in addition to her baby's pediatrician. He was in it up to his neck.

His strategy: get the mom and baby together in a controlled environment. She couldn't stay with her baby in ICU, and the hospital saw no reason to give them a room on the pediatric floor after the ICU treatment was complete. They were ready to send the baby home. Dr. Feinberg knew this wasn't safe. He insisted that the hospital should stay involved with psychiatric treatment of the mother, even if the baby's condition had stabilized.

After weeks of screaming to administrators, Dr. Feinberg received approval for his plan. The mother stayed with the baby on the pediatric floor under twenty-four-hour nurse observation. Now, the baby still stunk. Most of Dr. Feinberg's colleagues wouldn't even go into the room. But the mother's instincts and the lessons she had learned in therapy kicked in and overcame her psychiatric condition. She eventually went home with the baby. Nine years later, Dr. Feinberg still receives letters from the family, and still gets goosebumps as he reads them.

Trust on many levels was critical to the successful outcome of this case. The patient trusted the doctor enough to admit to something that would make most of us recoil in horror. The doctor trusted the patient enough to push for a treatment plan that would allow her to be with her baby in a controlled setting. The hospital finally learned to trust the doctor's judgment enough to rewrite the rules. This helped turn a potentially fatal situation into one where management and treatment could succeed. All of the players established a human connection. That allowed Dr. Feinberg to see how he could change the entire trajectory of his patients' lives. That sort of thing makes our jobs worthwhile.

Every doctor has a host of touching, life-changing stories like these. They don't happen every day, but even a few of them will keep her in the business. It's easy to see why just about anyone would be affected by needy patients—compassion is a basic human instinct. But for a doctor it goes beyond just feeling sympathetic to someone. Once the elements of trust, compassion, and information start to fall in place, your doctor is *empowered*. You can give her something that managed care has taken away. And you can do it without surrendering your own power to participate in mutual decisions about your treatment.

There are very simple ways patients help. In the next chapter, we will get into the territory that's most unfamiliar to patients—giving the doctor information. But first, we will concentrate on building trust and compassion. There are a few very simple dos and don'ts:

- Take care not to approach the relationship from a position of distrust. We are seeing more and more patients who demand an interview before visiting a doctor. If you think you need one, and can get one, fine. But during the interview, you want to be sure that he knows you are trying to build trust, not working from a position of distrust.

- If you are getting a second opinion, let your doctor know. Otherwise, out of the blue, he will get a request from Dr. Down-the-Road asking for your records. He won't know if you are out shopping or if you are just getting more information. Doctors don't mind when patients get second opinions. In difficult cases, it's better for them anyway.

- Don't expect your doctor to know who you are when you call. Saying "Hi, this is Jack" won't allow your doctor to tell you from Jill. There's no telling how many patients are on his roster. Give him more information: "This is John Patient, you saw me for [condition] on Tuesday and gave me [prescription or treatment]. You asked me to call back to let you know how it worked."

- Try to answer the questions as directly as possible. If you're asked a yes or no question, give a yes or no answer. Your doctor is trying to figure something out. Try to stay on the topic at hand. In the next chapter, we will show you a method for keeping the office visit focused.

- Don't tell him the real reason you came in at the end of the visit. So many patients wait until they're getting dressed before they tell doctors the real reason they came in. "By the way, can you get me on disability?" or "Say Doc, can you write me a Viagra prescription?" The reason you came in should be stated right at the start. If you act like you are hiding something, you've undermined trust.

- Don't expect your doctor to know information that you gave in the questionnaire you filled out in the waiting room. The same goes for information that you think is in your chart. If he asks you a question, he doesn't know. Don't refer him to your chart or become impatient, but try to answer the question.

- Don't expect a "two for one." Once patients have their doctors' attention, they tend to want to use it. Please don't ask your doctor to examine your child after he's done with you just because your child is with you. Don't expect him to give you advice on your uncle's chest pains. Make a separate appointment for your child. Encourage your uncle to seek treatment.

- Always be good to support people. The main nurse and secretary are closer to your doctor than you are. If you treat them like dirt, your doctor will hear about it. It's your reputation that will be soiled. Talk to them. Listen to their life stories. Bring them little gifts like cookies to brighten their day. Make them look forward to your next visit.

- Ask for help. Bring out that compassion. "I need your help. Can you help me?" works far, far better than "I want service" or "Are you just trying to keep costs down?"

By asking for help, being the kind of patient a doctor wants to help, and giving the information that allows him to help, you have sent the doctor a clear message: "You can now do what you were trained to do. You can be a doctor again." In this chapter, we have pulled back the curtain to let you see what forces are at work behind the cursory care we often get. We've given you insight into what makes the medical mind work. And we've shown you what you can do to make that mind work for you.

The next step is key. How to bring it all together in ten minutes or less. By building the stage with trust, and setting it with compassion, you are now ready to learn how to star in the production of this one-act medical drama. You are ready to learn how to give your doctor information.

When he was in medical school, your doctor learned a method for getting information from patients. He practiced this method until it was second nature. Then, in the real world, he found that patients don't always follow the plan. We are about to pull back the final curtain. Don't worry—this is a simple outline that anyone can learn. Just having a basic understanding of how he learned to diagnose will allow you to give him a problem to solve, a patient to care about, and the information he needs. By the time you are done, your doctor will feel like he's the one calling the shots, not the HMO. You'll both reap the benefits of the improved relationship.

~ 3 ~
The Ten-Minute Office Visit

QUESTIONS THIS CHAPTER ANSWERS

◆ How can I get great care in ten minutes or less?
◆ How can I use the HEAD (history, exam, assessment, decision) method?
◆ How can I get my doctor's attention?
◆ How do I describe my symptoms?
◆ What happens during an exam?
◆ How do doctors make diagnoses?
◆ How can I help develop a treatment plan?

Say you're driving to work one day and you hit a pothole. Everything seems fine at first, but then you notice the car shaking as you apply the brakes. The problem is still there when you drive home. You call the mechanic. He says he can squeeze you in, so you make an appointment to drop off the car the next day.

You're in a hurry when you come in, and the mechanic's obviously rushed, so you get right to the point. "I hit a pothole, there's a clanging noise, the car shakes when I stop." You're out in less than two minutes. You know better than to waste his time and yours by going over every minor problem the car has ever had—the dashboard lights don't work, the paint is peeling, the windshield wiper fluid is low. You don't tell him that your uncle had a similar problem with his car nor do you complain that you heard something on TV about how bad potholes have gotten in the city because of the lack of money for road repairs. On the other hand, you don't expect the mechanic to figure out the problem for himself. We seem to know how to get to the point in situations like this.

It's amazing how rarely this happens between doctors and patients.

A patient who comes in for a headache can suddenly start wandering all across his medical history. Suddenly the doctor is confronted with the sinus headaches the patient had as a child, the mole on his left leg, and how his uncle died from food poisoning. At the other extreme are patients who get right to the point, but then can't get past it. They say they have a headache, but when asked where, when, and how bad, they say, "I'm not sure. I don't have one right now. Is that important?"

We are not our cars. We aren't emotionally wrapped up in our cars' problems. We aren't intimidated by mechanics. We know that our cracked windshield isn't related to the shaky brakes. But faced with a medical problem and a doctor, we can easily develop high anxiety about every pain, twitch, or discomfort that we experience. We might be nervous and forget what we wanted to say, or clam up because of fear. We might have so much faith in our doctor that we think all we have to do is sit there, let him examine us, take his tests, and pull a diagnosis out of his pocket.

This might have worked in the old days when doctors had time. This is no longer true. A typical office visit today in managed care is just ten minutes. That's ten minutes to make introductory conversation, take the patient's history, do a physical exam, come to a diagnosis, and make a plan. The clock is ticking and every second counts. Every irrelevant fact, unwarranted concern, or unanswered question eats into your time. There has to be a choreographed give-and-take that can only happen in a mutual relationship.

But how can we tell which facts are relevant and which questions the doctor will ask? She's the one with the medical degree, after all. She's the one trained to find out what's wrong with you and what to do about it. That's true, but she doesn't feel your pain. She isn't experiencing your discomfort. Without your help in the form of exact descriptions of what you are going through, she will never get to an answer.

When your doctor was in medical school, she learned a method for getting all of the relevant information she needs to make a diagnosis. She spent years practicing on patients under close supervision. She learned that each office visit should be conducted using a standard plan with four steps. In a general practitioner's forty-year career, she might go through these steps 200,000 times. We are about to teach you these steps. If you are ready to explain your problem using this template, her job becomes as easy as filling out a form. Having saved both time and effort by following this routine with you, your doctor will have the chance to really get excited about making you well.

The beauty of this approach is that it has three effects, all of which lead directly back to you and your health. First, your doctor will see that you are cooperative, concerned, and ready to work with her as a partner. You will be the sort of patient who makes her day. Second, you will get her attention. Giving her all the information she needs, in the order she learned to take it, will remind her of the days when doctoring was about working with the patient and solving his problems. Third, you will master the ten-minute office visit. You will find that for most problems, ten minutes is all you really need to get the care you deserve. All you need to learn are the four stages of the office visit. All you have to remember is the word HEAD.

History

Exam

Assessment

Decision

We will take you through each of these steps in detail, giving you a "script" of what to say and when to say it. Perhaps even more important, we will give you pointers on what *not* to say. This format will work for any doctor, and for any ailment. It might take a little practice, but when you master HEAD, you will have mastered managed care.

HEADs Up: Getting Ready for Your Visit

We don't tend to be very organized when we go to the doctor. Instead, we are preoccupied with worries about what we will say, what she might find, or what uncomfortable procedures we will have to undergo. The result: we show up completely unprepared. It's a strange way to act. When we have a job interview or a business meeting, we might be anxious, but we prepare anyway. We know what we are going to say, we think about the questions we want to ask, and what will be asked of us. We get ready to build a mutual relationship with our interviewer or client.

And as we prepare for a business meeting, our worries start to fall away. If worries come up again, we just repeat to ourselves what we have practiced. The visit to your doctor shouldn't be so different. Getting ready can help you relax. Organizing your thoughts will keep anxiety at bay. Once you are in the examining room, your organization will allow the doctor to take a direct route to a diagnosis.

So instead of rushing off to your appointment, take time to prepare. Think about your problem, where it hurts, what might have caused it, and how you are going to communicate your symptoms to your doctor.

Let's say you are going to the doctor because you have diarrhea. It's gross. It's the last thing you want to think about, much less look at. But you will have to put that aside for a moment and give it some serious thought. Your doctor will want to know about this unpleasant bodily function in detail. When did the diarrhea start? How many times per day have you needed to use the bathroom? Is your stool bloody? Watery with no form? Does it float? What color is it? Have you started any new medicine recently? Had any foreign travel in the past few weeks?

If your doctor knows the answers to these and other questions, he can begin to pinpoint exactly where in your digestive system the problem lies. If he doesn't, he will waste valuable time trying to get the answers. Even worse, he might have to (perhaps unnecessarily) send you off for a stool sample. You can make your visit efficient and possibly avoid unnecessary tests with some simple planning.

The same can be said of other, less sensitive problems. Before you reach for the aspirin, think about how your headache feels. Is it throbbing? Sharp? Radiating? Is your scalp tender? What time of day does it happen? Is there a pattern? Are there other things affected by the headache, such as your vision? Thinking about these things before you go to the doctor will keep you from searching for the answer as your time runs out.

We are about to give you an organizational tool for thinking about your problems. It's the same tool your doctor learned when he was a medical student, but don't worry, it isn't hard to follow, and will easily become second nature because it makes sense. We've also provided a form in appendix A for you to photocopy and fill out before your visit. Taking the time to do this will ensure that you get all the care and attention you need in ten short minutes. In addition, there are a few other things you can do before you leave for the doctor's office:

- Think about what sort of questions your doctor might ask.
- If you haven't already given him your past medical history, or if you are changing doctors, write down what has happened to you in the past. Dates are very important.
- Put all your prescription and over-the-counter medicines in a plastic bag. Take it with you.
- Rehearse what you are about to say.
- Take a deep breath, and you are ready to go.

We are about to show you the "exhaustive" medical history. You might wonder how this could possibly fit into ten minutes. Don't

---

GETTING THROUGH THE HISTORY—SOME GENERAL TIPS

- Make eye contact. Your doctor may walk into the room with his head buried in a chart. Wait until you can make eye contact before you start talking.

- Always go from general to specific. This is how the doctor has been taught to think.

- Always go from subjective (what you feel) to objective (information you can see, count, or touch). Your doctor's thought is also moving in this way.

- Always explain how your problems affect your life, work, relationships, sleep, etc. This will help bring out the doctor's compassion, help her realize she's treating a person, not just a disease.

- Pause between parts of the history. This will allow your doctor to take notes and ask questions.

- A note on notes: Just because your doctor is scribbling frantically doesn't mean he's not listening. It's actually a good sign that he can use what you are telling him. On the other hand, he might not take notes while you are talking about sensitive subjects. Don't worry, he's just being sympathetic.

- Don't expect reassurance. Your doctor won't say "It's going to be okay" or "I'm sure it's nothing" until she is sure. She wouldn't want to reassure you only to have to break bad news later.

worry; as you bring your doctor to focus on your current problem, many of the items we are about to discuss will become unnecessary. Both you and your doctor will be in a position to judge what needs to be left out. If you are prepared and organized, however, you will be amazed at how much ground you can cover in just a few minutes.

"H" Is for History

This is where it all begins. The history is the first step toward a plan, and by far the most important. The history is the patient's chance to explain in his own words what the problem is. The patient's words are the key. Studies of how doctors diagnose have shown that between 60 and 70 percent of all the information they need comes from the history.

Managed care means that the history is even more important than ever. Since tests cost money, doctors can't rely on them like they used to. The history, on the other hand, is free. Doctors are being encouraged and trained to take all they can from the patient's own statements, following the advice of Sir William Oster, given back in 1905: "Listen to the patient. He is telling you the diagnosis."

As a patient, you can make it even easier to allow the doctor to extract a diagnosis from your own words. He's filling out a form while

---

THE PARTS OF THE MEDICAL HISTORY

Identifying data

Source of referral (if any)

Source of history

Chief complaint

Present illness: location, quality, quantity or severity, timing, setting, factors, and associated symptoms

Past health

Current health

Family history

Social history

Review of symptoms

you talk—if not a paper form, then one in his mind. Think about how much easier it would be for him if you just followed the form. There's no big medical mystery behind the file he's holding in his hands. It's a simple matter of classifying and separating data. Take a minute to absorb the outline of the medical history that appears as a sidebar. We'll then take you through each step.

We're going to help you by providing the approximate time each stage of the office visit should take, along with a running total. Don't worry about sticking to these times exactly. Some conditions—a neurological problem, for example—will require a shorter history and a longer exam. Use the times as guidelines, but be ready to put them aside if your doctor needs more time for a particular question.

Identifying Data: Who Are You?

Time: 10 seconds

When the doctor walks in, your history has begun even before either of you say hello. Figuring out who you are is the first step to figuring out what's wrong. You may have filled out a form in the waiting room that asked you, among many other things, your age, sex, occupation, and marital status. You may assume that the doctor has read this and fully absorbed it. But remember, this is managed care. You can't assume anything.

So when the doctor walks in, smiles, and asks what's wrong, the proper response is to first say who you are. This includes:

- Age
- Ethnic background
- Place of birth
- Marital status
- Occupation
- Religion
- Sexual preference

Giving the doctor your identifying information calls attention to yourself. It lets the doctor know exactly who he is dealing with, and could contain clues about what may be causing your problem. This is how doctors talk to each other about patients. Rather than saying, "I'm treating a diabetic," they always start out with identifying information: "I'm treating a fifty-six-year-old white, married, retired male who has diabetes."

Some of the items in the list above are very personal. We know this, and we know you may feel uncomfortable offering this information. You may wait for the doctor to ask. That's not the way to get the best care.

We know a female OB-GYN who treated a woman for fifteen years. The doctor would routinely ask the patient what sort of birth control she was using. The doctor would sometimes become concerned about her patient, who insisted she wasn't trying to get pregnant, and give her condoms and literature on STDs. Finally, the woman one day said, "Look, I know you are just trying to help, but I'm celibate." The patient was actually a little ticked off about getting all these questions about sex, but the doctor had to ask. The doctor, of course, was embarrassed and regretful for having made an incorrect assumption. But she also knows that she couldn't have done anything differently. The result was a strained relationship after fifteen years of cooperation.

The doctor *needs* to know some personal things about you for very important reasons. Being honest and open from the beginning about sexual orientation may save your life later. It also has the secondary effect of gaining the doctor's respect. A doctor is more likely to appreciate your honesty than judge you for your beliefs and practices.

Your religion also tells your doctor something about how you should be talked to, what procedures you might object to, and how you view illness. Here again, you will not be judged, except as a cooperative and honest patient.

Your ethnic background tells the doctor what diseases you may be at risk for. People of southern Italian descent are more likely to have beta thalasemia. People of African descent are more likely to have sickle cell anemia. The same goes for your place of birth. For example, multiple sclerosis only occurs in people born in northern latitudes. If you don't tell your doctor your ethnic background or place of birth, especially if you are mixed-race, he may not look down the right avenues or may waste time barking up the wrong tree.

If you need confidentiality about your sexual orientation or religion, be sure to say so. A doctor can make a mental note without entering this information on your chart. Just let him know that you would prefer not to have a record of the sensitive information you have just told him. But always place your health above your need for confidentiality.

Try different ways of delivering your identifying data until the information rolls off your tongue:

> "I'm a forty-two-year-old black heterosexual divorcee. I work as a stockbroker. I was born in Costa Mesa, California, and I'm a Christian."

> "I'm a gay white female. I was born twenty-nine years ago in Ogden, Utah, but left after I was laid off at the newspaper five years ago. I now work as a marketing executive at a radio station. I don't belong to any organized religion."

It takes less than ten seconds to lay your life out on the table. Once you have covered the basics, be sure to mention any recent life changes. Tell the doctor if you have recently moved, changed jobs, been married or divorced, or had children. Any life change can contribute to, aggravate, or relieve illness. Where you are in life, and how you feel about it, can affect your physical well-being. Even if you have told the doctor nothing that will help her with a diagnosis, you have presented yourself as a *person*, not just a patient. That can get even the busiest doctor focused and motivated.

Source of Referral: Who Sent You?

Time: 2 seconds   Running time: 12 seconds

After you tell the doctor who you are, he will want to know who sent you. He knows something about you in the wider world, now say where you are in the medical world: "I was referred to you by my PCP, Dr. Firststop." "I was self-referred." "A coworker who's on the same plan recommended you."

Doctors rarely get this kind of information directly from patients. And just like any other professional, they like to know why someone has come to their door. If the doctor has a connection with the referring person, you may get extra-special attention. It also helps the doctor answer the next question: Where can I learn more?

Source of History: Where Can I Learn More?

Time: 2 seconds   Running time: 14 seconds

The first source of a history is always you. But who else has asked you these questions? Does another doctor or hospital have a history on you? Did you fill out a form in the lobby? Do you have a referral letter from another doctor? If so, this is the time to pull it out: "My records can be found at the Hospital of Health in Wellsville, Arkansas." "I have this referral letter from Dr. Seeyalater."

Identifying data, source of referral, and source of history give your doctor enough of a background to start attacking the problem. Now it's time to present him with your problem.

Chief Complaint: Why Are You Here?

Time: 6 seconds   Running time: 20 seconds

Time to get down to brass tacks and explain, in brief summary, what made you decide to come in—your *chief complaint*. The emphasis is on *chief*. You may have other problems. You may already be getting treatment for other problems. But here you want to get the doctor to focus on the one problem that is most important to you right now.

As we mentioned in the last chapter, you can really push your doctor's buttons by waiting until you are on your way out before you say why you came in. Doctors call this the "doorway question," and patients are notorious for springing it. Now we hope you can see why it drives them crazy. After he has spent the exam addressing why the patient came in, the doorway question tells the doctor he was off-track the entire time. In a perfect world, the only ethical thing to do would be to call the patient back and do the exam over. But there are other patients to see, and so the only practical thing to do is attempt to salvage the history with the patient out of the room. It's nearly impossible to do the job right under these conditions, so be sure to give the *real* reason you came in at this stage.

Remember that the chief complaint is a summary. You will get to spend more time on the problem at the next stage of the history. The form the doctor is filling out encourages him to phrase the chief complaint in the patient's own words, so speak to the point.

"I have a stomach pain that started three days ago, it won't go away, and I'd like to figure out what the problem is."

"I have chronic low back pain that's gotten much worse in the past eight months. I can't work and I'd like to get on disability."

"I'm seeing a discharge from my penis that has me concerned. It started one week ago. "

You may not have a specific complaint. In that case, try to phrase your reason for coming in as a goal. Doctors will be very pleased to hear this.

"I'm coming in for my annual check-up despite feeling great."

"I've been told that I should be concerned about heart disease and would like a thorough evaluation."

"I'm here for my recommended 'well-woman' exam."

"I'm trying to get pregnant."

If you've followed each step so far, you have gone from zero to sixty in about twenty seconds. It's time to pause. You doctor at this point may want to start asking specific questions. He may be so surprised at having a patient who tells him everything he will need to know that he needs a moment to pick his jaw up from the floor. In just a few seconds, however, it will be time to move onto a thorough description of your symptoms. This next step will be the one where your clarity, organization, and preparation will bring the doctor more than half-way to a diagnosis.

Present Illness: Where, When, Why, and How Does It Hurt?

Time: 1 minute 10 seconds   Running time: 1 minute 30 seconds

When we feel pain and discomfort, it's all our own. It's very difficult to make someone understand what we are going through. That's why, at this stage of the history, doctors follow a specific set of questions to get to the root of the problem. Each subtle detail about your symptom is a clue that will lead your doctor to a diagnosis. It's vitally important to be honest, detailed, and exact at this stage of the history. That's why we recommended, earlier in this chapter, that you think long and hard about your symptoms before you come in. Now we are about to show you how your doctor thinks about symptoms.

Each symptom has a particular location, quality, quantity or severity, timing, setting, factors, and associated symptoms. These are the terms your doctor uses to describe the what, where, when, and how of your symptoms. It will be helpful to take some time with each of these ways of explaining your situation.

Location

This is always the best place to start. You will want to be specific, and even point to the affected area. If it's a widespread pain, you might want to draw a circle with your finger around the problem area. Speak while you do this: specify with your voice whether it's on your left side or right side while you demonstrate with your finger. Does the pain spread? If so, start where it seems to be centered, and show where it travels.

Sometimes symptoms aren't *felt* in a specific location. In these cases—blurred vision, bloody urine, diarrhea, for example—replace "where" with "what." Tell him what you have noticed. If you have *ever* felt any physical discomfort along with these symptoms, be sure to give the location of those sensations as well.

Quality

How does it feel? If we're talking about a discharge, how would you describe it? What does it look like? What does it smell like? If the problem is in your mouth, what does it taste like? The quality of a symptom can be a difficult thing to express, so try to use as many senses—sight, touch, taste, smell, hearing—as apply to your situation.

Is your pain shooting, stabbing, piercing, throbbing, pressing, gnawing, or pounding? Be creative. It's not medical terminology, but it's okay to say you feel like you have a ton of bricks on your chest. If it feels like you are being pricked by a thousand needles, say so. A diagnosis always moves from the subjective (what you feel) to the objective (what your doctor can see, feel, or measure). This is the time to be subjective.

What do you see? Do you see spots? Stars? Do you have blind spots? Blackouts? If it's a cut or sore that's become infected, what color is it? What color is the discharge coming out of it? If the problem is diarrhea, what color is that? If you have a rash, what shade of red is it? Is it on the surface or just below the skin? Are there blisters? If you have a chance to look at your problem, take a close look, and tell the doctor what you see.

What do you smell? Do you smell odors that seem to come from nowhere? Does the infected cut have an odor? Does the diarrhea or urine have an odor? What does it smell like?

Do you hear anything? Does your stomach growl while you are having abdominal pain? If your problem is in your joints, do they creak? Snap? Crackle? Pop? Grind? If your problem is associated with breathing, have you listened to yourself breathe? Is there whistling? Wheezing? Gurgling?

Talking about one's personal experience with a symptom can be a difficult task. To get your message across, feel free to use as many adjectives as you think are appropriate. Try to approach the chief complaint using as many senses as you have available. The result may sound vague, but your doctor has been trained to take clues even from these subjective statements. And besides, the next step will move us into more concrete territory.

Quantity or Severity

When doctors ask for lab tests, they are looking for hard numbers to test their first impressions. It's the way science works—you go from an experience or perception that's unique to a calculation that can be shared. This is what you are doing when you go from talking about the quality of your symptom to the quantity or severity of your symptom. You have crossed into objective territory.

Try being an amateur scientist. If your problem lies in shortness of breath, count how many stairs you can climb before you start to gasp for air. If you've experienced your symptom while exercising, how long before you have to stop? How many pages can you read before your headache kicks in? Take note of these things as they happen, but don't carry the experiment too far, and don't let your fact-finding aggravate your condition.

If your problem involves discharge, how much is involved? If you are having trouble urinating, how much are you able to get out? Just enough to fill a thimble? Or a cup? If it's a discoloration on your skin, how big is it? The size of a quarter? Or the size of a saucer? If your problem is related to menstruation, how often do you change your tampon or pad? When you do, is it lightly spotted or soaked? Numbers, even if they're just best guesses, are fuel for the medical mind. Your doctor can use them to start framing the picture you painted with your description of the symptom's quality.

If you don't have numbers ready, think about how else you can be objective. How severe is the problem? Compare it to something else. Perhaps your current headache is worse than the sinus headaches you had as a child, but not as bad as the time you had a concussion. Maybe your abdominal pain isn't as bad as heartburn, but is worse than hunger. Using a scale between zero (none) and ten (the worst possible) can help a doctor put the issue in perspective.

It's also extremely helpful to tell the doctor how this problem has affected your life: "It's so bad I can't have sex with my husband." "I've been able to go to work, but I can't lift heavy objects by myself." "I can't play with my kids." These sorts of statements aren't numbers, but they explain your problem *objectively*. They also have another, even more important effect. They allow your doctor to see *you*, and not just the symptom. They tell him how your problem has changed your life. They bring out his compassion and empathy.

Timing

Now that you've framed your condition more objectively by describing it in terms of quantity and severity, the next issue to discuss is its timing. When did your problem start? How long does it last? How frequently does it occur? Start at the beginning. When did you first experience this problem? From there, tell a story. Give a brief account of how it's changed, when it's happened since then, and when it happens now.

The more exact you can be, the better. If you haven't been watching the clock when you experience your symptoms, take your best guess. Tell the doctor, for example, that it lasts from midmorning to early afternoon, or from the time you get home until the time you go to bed. If you've noticed a pattern, you have noticed something very important. Don't forget to share it with your doctor.

Setting

Where were you and what were you doing when this problem first came up? If it's a recurring symptom, where are you and what are you doing when it goes away and comes back? What emotions are you feeling when it happens? Who are you with? What sort of things are in the place where it happens? Bright lights? Fumes? Sawdust? Pets? Describe the locations where the problem comes up. Then explain what you were doing there. Next, explain what you were feeling: "The last time it happened was when I was at work and the boss yelled at me. I thought I was going to lose my job." "The first time I noticed it was after playing softball. I hit a home run that won the game, but after the celebration, my shoulder hurt."

By giving the doctor the setting in which the symptom occurs, you are pointing him in the direction of external factors that might have caused your problem. Giving your symptom a general background allows you both to move onto the next phase of describing your symptom: what factors do *you* know of that make it better or worse?

Factors

Think closely about what makes your condition change. It might change for the better, or for the worse, or it might just change in quality. For example, it might change from a throbbing pain to a sharp pain. What makes it change? Try to put the factors in the settings you have just described. Here again, you are going from the general to the specific, following the train of thought that your doctor learned in medical school.

A factor can be anything: a person, activity, food, drug, drink, or emotion. You might think of a factor that seems ridiculous to you, but don't leave it out! This is one of the most important clues to solving your problem. Factors speak *directly* to a cause and a cure.

Does it hurt less when you lie down? Or does it get worse? Does exercise make it better? Does eating make it go away or make it worse? What foods make it better or worse? Does it get worse when you are nervous or angry? Does it get better when you are happy? Does it get better or worse when certain people are around? Have you tried any herbal remedies or over-the-counter medications that caused any change? Don't forget to mention any illegal drugs, if you use them. Do they make it better or worse? How so?

Once you have gotten through this step, you have completely described your chief complaint. Your doctor has almost everything he needs. He now knows where the problem is, what it's like, how bad it is, how often it happens, and what might cause it or cure it. He's already thinking of a treatment. The very last step in describing your symptom will encourage your doctor to expand his thinking. He already has an idea of what it might be, now you can give him a chance to think of what *else* it might be.

Associated Symptoms

At the beginning of this chapter, we compared your body to a car. You wouldn't tell your mechanic every small thing that's wrong with your car. You just want the main problem fixed.

The truth about your body, of course, is that it's much more complicated. That's why we doctors need the template of HEAD to organize the data we get from patients. We don't recommend that you ignore your minor symptoms, but we do recommend that you tell your doctor about them *after* you have fully described your chief complaint. It's just a way to save time and keep the doctor focused.

Now that you have described your chief complaint, think about what else you experience. The parts of your body are delicately linked. It's pretty rare that one part can be affected without affecting another part. If your doctor knows what else is affected, he can start looking at the whole illness, and not just the chief symptom.

Dr. Theodosakis recalls a patient, George, who came in for an evaluation of finger pain. His fingers were the only thing bothering George at the time. Through detailed questioning, Dr. Theodosakis learned that George had experienced an eye infection a few days earlier. George had also felt some minor burning while urinating but this had ceased for the most part. Dr. Theodosakis immediately recognized that the finger pain was due to a treatable form of arthritis (Reiter's) caused by a sexually transmitted bacterial infection, something that would probably have not been considered without knowledge of the associated symptoms. When Dr. Theodosakis asked about the patient's sexual history, sure enough, he found that weeks before, George had become sexually active with a new partner.

Say your chief complaint is a high fever. What other problems have you experienced? They might be so small that you wouldn't even consider going to the doctor for them alone. Do you have headaches with your fever? A minor pain in your side? Discoloration of your skin? A slight cough? General aches?

Any doctor will know what symptoms to ask about after you have finished with your chief complaint. But in managed care, in the space of a ten-minute office visit, these questions might get pushed aside. If you've been following HEAD, however, you've only used up a few of your ten minutes. You've given the doctor time to do his job right.

And when you list your associated symptoms, you've made his job more exciting. Fever alone isn't a very challenging problem for a doctor to solve—he's seen it hundreds of times. Most of the time the prescription is pain killers and rest. He might not even bother to figure out what's causing the fever until and unless it gets worse. But when you start to list associated symptoms, you are handing him a puzzle to solve. He can't keep himself from reconsidering his initial plan. That's what he was trained to do.

Give your doctor an associated symptom and see what happens. If he wants to know more, describe that symptom just the way you described your chief complaint. Then see if he asks you about other related symptoms. If you have more, offer them and describe them in the way you have learned. In the end, you might have nothing more than a simple problem. But you've still managed to make your doctor's day a bit more interesting.

Pulling It Together

We've covered a lot of ground since we last checked our clock. By now you might be wondering how you can possibly go through the seven parts of your chief complaint in one minute or less. Relax, it's easy if you are organized and prepared. Before you visit the doctor, go over each way of describing a symptom. Apply each one to your chief complaint. Then put together what you have into a few sentences. Read it to yourself to make sure you haven't left anything out. You will be surprised at how quickly your symptom can be summarized. These examples cover everything we have recommended in the last few pages:

> "One morning a few weeks ago, while I was getting up from bed, I suddenly noticed a sharp, stabbing pain in my lower left back that radiated down my left leg to my calf. It got so bad that I couldn't bend over without making it worse. I've had it on and off since but it seems to go away at night when I lie down. Ibuprofen, which I take eight times a day, doesn't seem to help. Sometimes, I also get headaches right after the back pain flares."

> "I've had three periods in the last month, and they've been much heavier than normal. I've had to change my tampon six times a day, which disrupts my business meetings. I even had to take time off from work. The menses are full of clots and darker than usual. I also have excruciating cramps, lower back pain, and more bloating than normal."

> "I've been feeling fatigued ever since I started my new job six months ago. The hours aren't anything I'm not used to, but all I can do when I'm at home is sleep. I even started nodding off at my desk the other day. It's this all-over tiredness, and my head feels heavy. I feel okay in the morning, but by the time I get to work, I'm ready to collapse. I've stopped exercising, and I've increased my vitamin dosage, but nothing seems to help. Sometimes I also feel dizzy, like everything's far, far away."

Even the longest of these examples takes no more than thirty seconds to read out loud. That leaves plenty of time for the doctor to ask follow-up questions and for you to describe any associated symptoms. When you are done, you will be no more than two minutes into the ten-minute office visit. And look at how much you have accomplished: The doctor has the entire story of your chief complaint. You've wasted no time in getting to the root of the problem, and you've given him a challenge to work with. He's already thinking of possibilities. The rest of the visit will be devoted to refining and testing those possibilities. There's still more ground to cover, but you have given your doctor a roadmap and pointed him in the right direction.

Past Health: What's Happened Before?

Time: 30 seconds   Running time: 2 minutes

Now that your chief complaint has been covered, it's time to see if there are any clues in your past. Take note of when this part of the history is discussed—after your chief complaint is out on the table. Be sure you have said all you want to say about your current problem before you delve into your past.

The first thing you want to do is say whether your chief complaint has occurred before or not. This makes for a smooth transition. The doctor may want to take the lead in asking you questions about your past health. Let him. He knows what to look for. But if he doesn't, you can take the lead by covering these important topics:

- General state of health in the past. Be honest. Say how closely you monitor your health, and how often you see the doctor.

- Childhood illnesses. Chicken pox, pneumonia, meningitis, any others you can think of. Were you a premature baby?

- Adult illnesses. For now, just give the ones that are in the *past*. Were these problems solved to your satisfaction?

- Psychiatric conditions. Were you ever on Prozac? Have you ever been admitted to a psychiatric hospital? Have you ever felt suicidal? How were the problems resolved?

- Accidents and injuries. Have you had any broken bones? Have you ever been knocked unconscious? Any severe cuts or lacerations? Any food, chemical, or drug poisoning? Was the problem resolved?

- Any operations or hospitalizations? Be ready with the doctor's name, the hospital, and the name and date of the operation. Some patients don't mention plastic surgeries, but even liposuction and tummy tucks are important. So are cesarean sections.

Each of the above questions can almost always be addressed in a single sentence, so even if you answer all of them you will be adding only a few seconds to your running time. Next, you will want to be prepared to answer questions about your current health.

Current Health: How Are You?

Time: 30 seconds   Running time: 2 minutes 30 seconds
This section of the history is a different from "associated symptoms," which you covered just seconds earlier. For example, if you have asthma but came in for shoulder pain, you wouldn't list asthma as an associated symptom—it's one that you live with regardless of your current condition. But it could be very important. The drugs you are taking for asthma might be causing your current condition. The drugs the doctor prescribes might interact with your asthma medication. So it's very important to summarize your current health. Get yourself ready for the following questions:

- Do you have any allergies? Do you have hay fever? Are you allergic to penicillin or other medications?

- What immunizations have you had? Flu shots? Tetanus? Childhood immunizations?

- What screening tests do you have regularly? Physical exams? Blood tests? Chest X rays? TB skin tests? Electrocardiograms (EKGs)? Brain scans? Pap smears? HIV (AIDS) screening?

- Are you HIV-positive? Many patients leave this out, fearing their doctors won't touch them. This will not keep the doctor from making contact. But it's something they *need* to know.

- Are you regularly exposed to hazardous chemicals? Spray paint? Solvents? Asbestos?

- How often do you exercise? What kind of exercise? How long? How many sessions per week?

- What else do you do with your leisure time?

- How well or poorly do you sleep?

- Do you follow any special diet? Low fat? Vegetarian? Do you eat a wide variety of fruits and vegetables? Do you skip meals? Restrict your food intake? Eat "diet" foods or formulas?

- Do you drink coffee, tea, or cola? Anything else with caffeine? Try to give typical amounts. If you take your lattes with a double shot, be sure to say so.

• Do you smoke? How much? For how long? Have you ever tried to quit? Try to estimate your total exposure to tobacco in your life in *pack-years*. One pack of cigarettes per day for one year is one pack-year; one-and-a-half packs per day for six years is nine pack-years. Knowing this number ahead of time is helpful.

• Illegal drugs. Always, always mention these, even if you aren't asked. Say what it is you take, how much, and how often. How potent are the drugs you take? How do you feel under the influence? If you have *ever* used needles to inject drugs, even years ago, you must add this to your history. Physicians are not required to document this type of information, so if you ask for confidentiality, there's a good chance your doctor won't enter it on your chart. If confidentiality is important for you, raise your concern at the same time you start talking about sensitive issues.

• What over-the-counter, prescription, and herbal drugs or supplements do you take? You will want to have these with you and be ready to answer the following questions: What is the name of the product? What is the dose? How many times a day do you take it? When did you start?

We can't emphasize this enough: *Bring your medicines with you.* If you can't, then bring an up-to-date, totally accurate list. Each year, there are over 135,000 hospitalizations and tens of thousands of deaths in this country due to adverse drug interactions. Even herbal drugs can interact with other drugs. Each one of these tragedies is preventable, but your doctor can't help you unless you show him what you are taking. There's no excuse for wasting time and jeopardizing your health by telling the doctor that you take a "little blue pill" and assuming he'll know which one (of hundreds) it could be.

You might not cover each item listed above, but you should be ready with a quick answer if the doctor asks. If, on the other hand, you suspect that any of the items above are related to your chief complaint, be sure to bring them up yourself. If you have made any recent changes—for example, in your diet, sleep pattern, or exercise regimen—be sure to bring these up. Always mention prescription, over-the-counter, and even illegal drugs.

If you and your doctor are selective with this section, and you are ready with your answers, it shouldn't take more than thirty seconds to complete your current health history. You are getting near the end of the history. Next up: What's happened in your family?

Family History: Is It in Your Genes?

Time: 30 seconds   Running time: 3 minutes

Most of the time you can be selective with this section. It might not even come up, or your doctor may ask specific questions. Still, there is information that you should volunteer, especially if you are seeing this doctor for the first time. This is something that might be prepared in advance if you can't rattle it off the top of your head or at a moment's notice. Think for a minute about the health of your immediate family members (we call them first- and second-degree relatives). You should be able to provide a brief health summary for each: "Dad is sixty-five, living, and has high blood pressure and gout. Mom died at age sixty-three from pneumonia. Brother, thirty-one, has migraine headaches and hepatitis. Sister is thirty-three and healthy. Maternal grandma died at age seventy-seven from a heart attack." Et cetera. Do not go into their symptoms, how the diagnoses were made, or their life stories. The doctor is solely interested in what inherited conditions may affect your health. If any of your family members have the following conditions, be sure to let your doctor know:

- Alcoholism
- Anemia
- Arthritis
- Cancer (type)
- Diabetes
- Drug addiction
- Epilepsy
- Headaches
- Heart disease
- High blood pressure
- Kidney disease
- Mental illness
- Stroke
- Tuberculosis

When you bring any of these up, try to see whether the doctor thinks there is a cause for concern. You can even ask him. If he wants to know more, you should be ready to tell him how the disease progressed in your family member, whether the problem was solved, and if so, how. He might not be able to use this information to address your chief complaint, but he may recommend screening tests to monitor the problem. This might require another visit. For now, you want to focus on your chief complaint.

Social History: How Do You Live?

Time: 30 seconds   Running time: 3 minutes 30 seconds

Remember the very first piece of information you gave your doctor? "Identifying data"—a brief statement of who you are and what you do. At this stage, the history has come full circle. Now is the time to give the doctor more information about your life. Now that you and he have covered your current medical problem in detail, you can both view your life with an eye toward finding out what's wrong.

You can let your doctor take the lead in asking questions about your social history. He doesn't need to know *everything*, and he will know what he is looking for. Be brief and concise, do not make judgmental statements or wander. But don't hide anything from him. He is asking for important medical information. This discussion can also be valuable in building a bond of trust between you and your doctor. This is another chance to get him to see you as a person, not just a disease.

There's a good chance your doctor is going to ask you about sex. It's time to put your shyness on the shelf. Medically speaking, sex is just as important as diet. Inability to have or enjoy sex might be tied to your chief complaint. It might give clues to what causes it. Even lack of sexual problems says something about your health. You might have left a sexual problem out of your list of associated symptoms, thinking that it was irrelevant. This was a big mistake.

There's only one more section of the history. That means that in less than five minutes the doctor will have been able to gather 60 to 80 percent of the information he needs to make a diagnosis. Together, you are mastering the ten-minute visit.

Review of Systems: What Else Is Going On?

Time: 1 minute   Running time: 4 minutes 30 seconds

Many doctors combine the review of systems with the exam, but the purpose of the review is very different from that of the exam. The review of systems gathers subjective information—the patient's own words and experiences. The exam attempts to uncover objective information—physical signs of illness—and triggers the patient's memory about signs and symptoms they may have overlooked in the chief complaint. So if your review is combined with the exam, be sure to keep providing information in your own words while the exam is going on.

Other doctors give patients the review of systems to fill out in the waiting room. This is fine, except for the things that a standard form might miss. While you are filling it out, think about what the form doesn't cover, and be prepared to bring these issues up when you get to the review part of the history.

The review of systems is your chance to mention that mole on your left leg that's been bothering you for a while, but which you've never sought treatment for. It might not get attention now, but bringing it up during the review rather than during the discussion of your chief complaint keeps the history focused.

As we are getting close to the exam, you will be handing off more control to the doctor. In the review of systems, there are so many systems to cover that it just isn't possible to go through each one in detail during a ten-minute visit. If you have a full physical exam (allowed by most managed care plans every year or two), your doctor is much more likely to spend time on the issues uncovered in the review of systems. But for right now, let the doctor focus on those systems that have seen a noticeable change or are related to your chief complaint.

The review of systems covers a broad range of issues. Generally, you should be answering according to what you've noticed in the past few days to weeks. There are plenty of questions for you to think about:

- General—This covers weight change, sleep, weakness, fatigue, fever, and recent infections.
- Skin—Do you have any rashes, sores, itching, color change, or changes in your hair or nails?
- Head—You might not have a headache now, but have you had even a slight one during the course of your illness? Have you been getting more headaches recently?
- Eyes—How's your vision? Have you had it checked lately? Are you wearing contacts to the visit? Do you produce tears excessively for no

apparent reason? Is your vision blurred? Do you see spots or specks? Have you ever had glaucoma or cataracts?

- Nose—Any sinus trouble? Hay fever? Nosebleeds? Frequent colds? Discharge? Itching that won't go away?

- Mouth and throat—Do your gums bleed? Is your tongue sore? Is your mouth dry? Do you have a sore throat or hoarseness frequently?

- Neck—Do you have swollen glands? Any pain or stiffness in your neck?

- Breasts—Any lumps, pain, or discomfort? Any discharge from your nipples? Do you do a regular self-exam?

- Respiratory system—Do you have a cough you can't shake? Any phlegm? What color and how much? Do you have wheezing? Have you ever had asthma, bronchitis, emphysema, pneumonia, tuberculosis, or pleurisy? Do you smoke?

- Cardiac system—Have you had any heart trouble, high blood pressure, or murmurs? Have you ever had rheumatic fever, chest pain or discomfort, palpitations, dyspnea, orthopnea, or edema?

- Gastrointestinal system—Do you have heartburn, nausea, vomiting, regurgitation, or indigestion? Any trouble swallowing? Is there blood in your vomit? Any change in your bowel movements? Any rectal bleeding? Black tar-like stool? Constipation? Any abdominal pain? Intolerance to any foods? Excessive belching or passing of gas?

- Urinary system—How often do you have to go? Has it changed? Any burning or pain? Dribbling? Loss of control?

- Genitals—Have you ever had a sexually transmitted disease? How was it treated? What is your sexual preference? Are you interested in sex? Are you satisfied with your sex life?

- Genitals, male—Any discharge from your penis? Any sores? Any pain in your testicles? Do you use condoms?

- Genitals, female—Are your periods regular? Have you experienced bleeding after intercourse? Do you experience premenstrual tension? How bad is it? How many pregnancies have you had, if any? How many abortions, if any? Any miscarriages? What form of birth control do you use, if any? Are you in menopause?

- Peripheral vascular system (circulation through extremities)—Do you have any leg cramps? Varicose veins? Clotting history?

- Musculoskeletal system—Do you have any pain in your muscles or joints? Any stiffness? Arthritis? Do any joints feel unstable?

- Neurologic system—Any tremors, tics, or involuntary motion? Numbness, paralysis, or loss of feeling? Weakness? Have you experienced any fainting, blackouts, tingling sensations, or seizures? Ever been knocked unconscious?
- Hematologic system—Do you bruise easily? Have you ever had a blood transfusion?
- Endocrine system—Are you excessively hot or cold? Do you produce excessive sweat? Are you excessively thirsty or hungry?
- Psychiatric—Have you experienced memory loss? Are you experiencing mood swings? Are you tense or nervous? Have you been depressed?

That's a lot to think about, but it's just a few examples of what your doctor has to think about in order to take a complete history. We've shared this list of questions with you to get you thinking about possible associated symptoms. You might be able to tick off "yes" answers to three or four of these questions. Any more than that, and you will probably need more than ten minutes. But three or four can easily be handled in the space of a ten-minute visit. And remember, even though you are trying to be a proactive patient here, you don't want to exercise too much control over this part of the history. Let the doctor ask his questions, and be prepared with the answers.

You've finished the history. Your doctor now has everything you can tell him. This means that the subjective part of the visit is done. It's time to relax and let your doctor do a physical examination.

"E" Is for Exam

Time: 2 minutes   Running time: 6 minutes 30 seconds

For about four minutes, you have held the floor, preparing the doctor for his exam. He will now attempt to find physical evidence of your chief complaint. He will be asking you questions while looking you over, but for the most part, this is now his show. It's time for you to get undressed.

After taking your vital signs—heart rate, blood pressure, respiratory rate, temperature—your doctor will be doing a review of systems in his mind as he goes through the exam. He will start with the head, just like the review did, and work his way down. He will touch you, smell you, look at you, and listen to your organs through his stethoscope. Earlier in this chapter, we asked you to try for a mutual relationship with your doctor, rather than to accept a paternal-type relationship. During the exam, however, you will benefit from giving the doctor control over the situation. This is one time when your relationship can be a little less than mutual.

You will know that this time has come to an end when he tells you that you can get dressed. Now you can, once again, start taking an

---

TIPS FOR GETTING THROUGH THE EXAM

- Get undressed quickly and without fussing. This is no time to be shy. If, however, you have a real problem being naked or wearing those flimsy gowns, it's okay to say so. You doctor can help put you at ease.

- It's better to not wear clothes with excessive buttons or shoes with lots of laces. These can take minutes to remove, cutting into your time.

- You doctor is looking for clues everywhere. Don't try to mask a hygiene problem like bad breath. It might tell him something. Don't dress up to come to the doctor's office, but just come as you are.

- It's okay to point things out during the exam that you mentioned during the history. Then let the doctor take a look in silence.

- Even if you are answering a question, don't talk when your doctor has a stethoscope anywhere on your body. The sounds you make are amplified through the stethoscope and the doctor can't hear a thing.

- While examining your abdomen, your doctor will touch you lightly at first, then deeply, trying to actually feel your internal organs. If you experience pain, let him know. It's an important clue.

- No one likes rectal, scrotal, or vaginal exams. That includes your doctor. Try to understand that he only does it when it's necessary. Try to be cooperative.

- If you have a fear of a certain test or procedure, like a fear of needles, it's important to say so. The doctor then has a chance to put you at ease. It's better than keeping it to yourself, only to jerk your arm away at the last minute or faint on the table.

- Gently guide your doctor to those systems that are most affected by your chief complaint. "This is what has me worried," you might say.

active role in the process of figuring out what is wrong. The best way to start is with a simple question: "What did you find?"

"A" Is for Assessment

Time: 1 minute   Running time: 7 minutes 30 seconds

Your doctor has been thinking over what to do about your problem from the moment he saw you. Each thing you have said, each poke with his finger or sound through the stethoscope, has been entered into his thought process. It is a process, even if it looks like magic. Patients typically see doctors come to conclusions so quickly that it appears instantaneous, but it is a process. Just like the history and exam, the assessment follows a defined structure. This structure is so ingrained in doctors' minds that it has become automatic. That doctors can draw conclusions so quickly has benefits and drawbacks.

As we saw in the last chapter, the HMO can affect a doctor's thinking. Since the thoughts that lead him to a diagnosis are so ingrained, he might not even realize how cost-cutting measures have altered his approach. That's why it is vitally important for you to understand how your doctor makes an assessment. With this understanding, you can guide him away from the HMO's influence and back to where his thought is unfettered.

Assessment has seven steps: identify problems, identify abnormalities, place them anatomically, identify possible causes, hypothesize, test hypothesis, and finally, put it into words. Many of these steps will be invisible to you, but if you can think like your doctor, you will be one step closer to a mutual relationship with him and even closer to a beneficial relationship with your HMO. Here is what he is doing. You don't have to perform these steps, just understand how they work.

First Step: Doctor Identifies Problems

This has already been done, and you were the source. The doctor takes what you have told him and makes a list. There may be only one or two problems on this list, or there may be a dozen. From what you have told the doctor, try to make a list of your own. When you hear a hypothesis, you will be ready to ask if it covers all of your symptoms, or if additional assessment is needed.

Second Step: Doctor Identifies Abnormalities

"Problems" are what you tell your doctor about, "abnormalities" are what he found during his exam. Again, we've gone from subjective to objective. Again, your doctor has made a list. If you asked him what he found when he was done with the exam, then you can make a list of your own. Some of the abnormalities will clearly match up with problems. An abnormal heart rate, for example, might match a complaint of chest pains. Other problems will not match abnormalities so clearly, except to your doctor.

Third Step: Doctor Places Abnormalities and Problems Anatomically

When your doctor goes through this step of the process, she is placing your complaints and her findings into *systems*. One problem might go into the cardiac system, another might belong to the neurologic system. Your doctor knows how these systems can affect each other. So her findings and your problems are being further related and matched.

You can make an attempt at matching problems through systems. You might not be able to see clearly how one system can affect another, but just thinking in terms of the systems of your body can help you understand the diagnosis the doctor is developing.

Fourth Step: Doctor Identifies Possible Process

Doctors next start thinking about what "process" is involved in the condition. Here, the information from your history comes into play. One possible process is toxic. If you told your doctor that you are exposed to harsh chemicals at work, she might be thinking of how these toxins could create your problems. Here are some of the possible processes your doctor is considering:

- Congenital—Was it present at birth and just recently symptomatic?
- Hereditary—Was a gene defect acquired from parents or relatives?
- Immunologic—Has the immune system been overly activated or suppressed? Is there inflammation as a result?
- Nutritional/metabolic—Is it a problem with the process of turning

nutrition into living matter? Is it due to a lack of, excess, or imbalance of proper nutrients?

- Neurologic—Is it caused by a problem with the brain, spinal cord, or nerves?
- Musculoskeletal—Is it due to joint, muscle, tendon, ligament, or other connective tissue diseases?
- Oncologic—Is it due to cancer?
- Degenerative—Are the affected organs breaking down or is this normal aging?
- Endocrinologic—Is it due to a problem with glands or hormones?
- Vascular—Does it involve the blood vessels?
- Traumatic—Is it related to an acute or chronic injury?
- Toxic—Is it related to a poison or toxin?

Once your doctor has your story and her findings, has placed them in systems, and has identified a possible process, she is ready to make a hypothesis.

Fifth Step: Doctor Develops a Hypothesis

The first thing the medical mind does in order to create a hypothesis is to select the most specific findings—the ones that most directly point to the underlying problem. You may have given a fever as your chief complaint, but if your doctor discovers a swollen liver during the exam, she will shift her focus to this finding. This doesn't mean that your chief complaint is being ignored. Her next step is to match her findings to your symptoms. You will want to ask questions until you understand how the finding she selected relates to your chief complaint.

Symptoms are experiences that patients feel, and that may or may not be due to disease. One symptom, in fact, can indicate dozens of diseases. To narrow this list down, your doctor eliminates those diseases from her list that don't explain most or all of your relevant complaints and her findings. This is called a "differential diagnosis." If you have ideas about what your condition could be, you may want to ask why one or the other explanation has been ruled out. Her answer will usually be simple: the disease you suspect doesn't explain this or that symptom.

Your doctor then selects the most likely explanation for your symp-

tom. A headache and fever are early symptoms of many things, including an Ebola infection, but unless you have traveled to central Africa
recently, this possibility can safely be ruled out. You doctor will be taking your age, race, gender, and environmental factors like your occupation into account. She will be asking herself, "What is the most likely
explanation for *this* person?" This is why explaining who you are and
what you do is so important.

The last thing she considers are life-threatening possibilities. She
should question her own first impressions of your illness, just to make
sure that she hasn't made a fatal miscalculation. Be very aware here!
This is a critical moment! Sadly, this is also the moment when HMO
time pressures and financial needs could endanger your health. An
inexperienced doctor trying to quickly move on to the next patient
might skip this step accidentally.

This is very frightening, but there's a simple way to avoid this potential problem. When you hear your doctor's hypothesis, the first thing to
do is ask: "What else could it be?" Don't act suspicious or probing, just
let your concern show through. Usually, it only takes this one question
to make the doctor's medical training kick in. It's always an appropriate question, one that your doctor should have asked herself.

At this stage of assessment, your doctor's fact-gathering and
thought processes have resulted in a hypothesis. But a hypothesis isn't
a diagnosis until it's been tested.

Sixth Step: Doctor Tests Hypothesis

By now your doctor may have a good idea of what is causing your
problem. But he will want to be sure. Testing can take many forms:
more history-taking, a more detailed physical exam, or lab tests. The
doctor might also send you home with a prescription and instructions
to monitor your condition. Here again, you will have to be alert. Has
the HMO limited the doctor's ability to run certain tests? Are time
pressures keeping the doctor from thoroughly testing his hypothesis?

If you suspect that this is the case, there are key questions to ask.
You want to maintain a mutual relationship by asking your doctor to
explain his reasoning. There are a number of questions that will force
him to reconsider, but without making him think you are one of his
pain-in-the neck patients:

- "What's the best way to test for this?" This question emphasizes *best*, not *cheapest* or most convenient.

- "What other tests are available?" By asking this question, you have expanded your doctor's thinking about your condition.

- "What will this test tell you?" It's always good to know what the doctor is looking for, and this question might get the doctor to think about what might have been an automatic response.

- "What happens if it's negative or positive?" By asking this question, you are getting the doctor to think about the next stage—making a decision.

If you know of a particular test or procedure that would be helpful, be very careful about how you ask for it. If the doctor writes down the words "patient requests" there's no doubt that the request will be rejected. The doctor has to request the procedure and have medical reasons for requesting it.

So instead of directly demanding or requesting the procedure, guide him to make the recommendation himself. You can say things like "I've heard that this new treatment might help. What do you think?" or "Do you think the plan will approve this test for my case? I'd feel a lot better if I could get one." These requests will work much better than walking into the room and saying, "I want an MRI."

Seventh Step: Doctor Puts the Hypothesis into Words

The final step of assessment is to put the hypothesis into words. Usually, these will be words that only another doctor can understand. Try to get your doctor to explain it to you in plain English. See if you can have him relate it to your symptoms. Work with him until you are sure you understand what he is thinking.

Doctors often use medical-speak as a defense mechanism. They don't like giving bad news, or they might be trying to keep their emotional distance. So don't get angry or frustrated with your doctor if everything that comes out of his mouth is gibberish. Express your concern, pay attention, and ask questions.

Dr. Feinberg remembers a time when he had to tell two parents that their son had schizophrenia. This is a disease with no cure, a disease that turns lives upside down. Dr. Feinberg attempted to mask his sadness over the situation with a bunch of medical jargon, explaining what was happening in the patient's nervous system, how treatments could lessen the effects, and how research is attacking the problem. He admits now that he was sending the worst kind of message. The father of the patient broke in to ask him a question that cut right through the jargon: "Doc, are you telling me that I should build a room out back?" Dr. Feinberg had to rethink his whole approach—these were *people* before him whose lives were about to change. "What I am telling you," he replied, "is that your son is never going to grow up the way you dreamed."

Ask a question that puts your condition in perspective. Ask a question that makes your doctor focus on you, not just your condition. By doing so, you will not only gain a partner for attacking your illness, you will move the office visit to the next stage, the decision.

"D" is for Decision: Making a Plan with Your Doctor

Time: 2 minutes 30 seconds   Running time: 10 minutes

Time to wrap up your visit. By now you should have told your doctor all of your concerns, understood her diagnosis, and convinced her that you are ready to be an active player in your treatment. The final step is to decide how that treatment will proceed. Think like an empowered patient: the doctor or HMO should not *dictate* the terms of your treatment to you. Now more than ever, you need to have a mutual relationship with your doctor.

First, have you understood your condition? Ask your doctor what you should expect. What symptoms will you experience if it improves? What symptoms should alert you that it's getting worse? Understanding how your disease is likely to progress is especially important for following up.

What else can you do to improve the treatment? Would changing your diet help? Should you start looking for a new job? Most doctors shy away from telling their patients how to live their lives. In most cases this restraint is appropriate, but if you say that you are willing to change your lifestyle to get well, your doctor will be ready to share her opinion. Your plan for treatment shouldn't stop with what medical science can offer.

If you have received a prescription for medications, be sure you understand what they will do. Always ask about side effects. What drugs or foods does your prescription interact with? Ask your doctor what other drugs you should avoid. If she is recommending tests, ask her exactly what she is testing for, and what that will tell her. Are there any dangers associated with the test? Do you need to do anything special to prepare for the test? For example, should you avoid eating or drinking before the test?

Establish a time period for following up. Will you follow up by phone or with another office visit? What problems might arise that would mean you should come in sooner? When you call, remind the doctor who you are, what your problem is, and that she wanted you to call. Then give her the information she had requested you give during the follow-up call.

You are almost ready to leave, but you have one more question: "Am I covered?" For the entire office visit, you have kept your HMO out of the room. You have kept your doctor engaged with your problem. You have done everything you can to keep her from thinking about cutting costs. Now that she is firmly on your side, it's time to discuss where you stand in relation to your HMO.

You might be covered for everything the doctor has prescribed. But how far will your plan go? Will there be a point where you should leave the plan for additional treatment or tests? How much will that cost? These are questions your doctor will now be ready to answer. She has done all she can for you, and you have her sympathy. You have been frank with her, and she will now be ready to be frank with you.

Her answers may lead to revisions in the plan you have just established. Run through your decision again, if necessary. Then it is time to leave. Don't forget to look the doctor in the eye, smile, and say "Thanks for your help." We need to be reminded that we have the power to help. That goes double for those of us working in HMOs.

Treatment plans are always fluid. They can be revised, stopped, or radically altered. So don't let your HMO off the hook just because you have been sent home with a plan. If it works, great. If it doesn't, you will have to be ready to return to your doctor and develop a new plan. We will discuss treatment plans in more detail in chapters 4 and 6.

What Have I Accomplished?

As you leave your doctor's office, think about what just happened. You have talked with your doctor in his own terms. You have taken control of your own health without taking away your doctor's power to help you. You got his attention, made him listen, and reminded him of why he went to medical school. You kept the HMO's need to cut costs out of the picture, and you did it in a way that will make your doctor grateful. You kept your doctor's schedule moving, something he will remember you for. And finally, you were able to think about your own problem in a new way.

The tools we have given you for getting through the ten-minute office visit shouldn't be put away now. They are tools for changing the way you think about your health. Even after you have mastered the ten-minute office visit, managed care will continue to make demands on you to anticipate your potential problems and, at times, find your own solutions. In coming chapters, we will show you how you can develop a program of prevention and screening that will allow you to become your very own health maintenance organization.

~ 4 ~

Building a Doctor-Patient Partnership

QUESTIONS THIS CHAPTER ANSWERS

◆ *How do I get through to problem doctors?*

◆ *When should I change doctors?*

◆ *How does the HEAD method make me a "good" patient?*

◆ *How do I work with my doctor to develop a treatment plan?*

◆ *How do I build a treatment team in the hospital?*

The details in the last chapter on the history, exam, assessment, and decision cover everything you need to know about what a good doctor is looking for as he learns about your condition. As you can probably see by now, doctoring is detective work. When you have your clues organized, ready, and available, most of your doctor's job is done. He won't have to search, and he won't have to guess at the right question.

Using HEAD will make your doctor's day easier, but that's not the main reason we are sharing it with you. Presenting your complaints in this format works to his benefit, but the office visit is all about you—your needs, your treatment, your plan. Getting the doctor to look at you, to really look at and listen to you, is the primary goal of HEAD. Whenever it seems that your visit isn't going exactly as planned, remember this one vitally important goal. If your doctor is looking, you are on the way to getting the best care possible from your health plan.

Unfortunately, you can't always count on your doctor to ask the right questions, or to really look at you, his patient. Dr. Feinberg remembers well how he learned this lesson. During his first week as an intern, he and another intern were sent to see a patient and take his history. The two spent an hour and a half going through the procedure we gave you in the last chapter. That's pretty normal for a beginner. As HEAD sinks into our heads, however, we doctors become much more efficient with this tool. When Dr. Feinberg and his colleague were done, however, they were asked to tell their teacher and a group of students what they had learned.

Their teacher got right to the point of the lesson: "What did you see?"

"We didn't really see anything," Dr. Feinberg answered, "because we didn't do the exam. We were told to just take a history."

The teacher kept pressing them, however, on what they saw, not what they heard. Finally, he sent the embarrassed pair back into the examining room to just *look* at the patient. They were shocked when they did. He had a case of advanced scleroderma, a disease that hardens the outer layer of the skin. The man's face was distorted into a mask, but the novice doctors, focused solely on taking a history, had literally never looked at him while he answered their questions.

This may seem like an oversight only a beginner would make, but think for a moment about this case in light of what you have learned about history-taking. What went wrong? First, the doctors never got the patient's chief complaint. They focused on getting every detail, except the most crucial one. The doctors didn't think to pursue the leads presented by the symptoms and irregularities in the patient's history to lead them to more direct questions. The patient didn't stop them or try to offer anything beyond what they asked. Above all, the patient didn't make the doctors look at him.

In managed care, doctors are often beginners all over again. They might not feel they have the time or patience to look at you, ask the right questions, or become involved beyond taking a few notes. They might gloss over important points, thinking they can just review your chart later. But your chart is in a stack of unread charts on the doctor's desk, and there's no telling when he will find the time to look at it thoroughly. There's no telling whether the information he needs will actually be there.

A doctor friend of ours told us about a time she was called into the ICU because a patient, who had an operation three days earlier to remove a small bowel obstruction, was short of breath. She found that he had pneumonia, and prescribed antibiotics. However, she also noted that the patient was delirious. While reviewing his chart, she found that none of the patient's five doctors had taken note of his alcohol consumption. Questioning the patient, she learned that he normally drank four or five large glasses of wine with dinner. He hadn't had any that evening. It turned out the patient was going through delirium tremens, a potentially fatal condition precipitated by the sudden cessation of alcohol intake. The patient and the five treating doctors who saw him forgot to get a social history. The doctors were all experienced, but hadn't really *looked* at the patient.

Your doctor has to look at you. You may not want him to see your gross sores or learn about your unhealthy habits, but he has to look at you and learn about you. Even if you have a problem doctor or a rushed office visit, *always* remember to get him to look at you, no matter what.

The information your doctor gains by looking gives him the power to make decisions, take on the HMO if necessary, and really enjoy his work. Once you and the doctor have mutual understanding and control, a treatment plan—the real reason you came in—will fall into place.

In a perfect world, HEAD will always work, even in managed care. Ninety percent of the doctors you meet will see and appreciate what you are trying to do. The other 10 percent, however, will require a little extra work and a bit more diplomacy. The important thing is that you don't give up.

We are about to discuss these difficult cases and explain how you can still get through to your doctor. There are plenty of tricks and strategies for each type of doctor, but only one thing you should always keep in mind if you meet a difficult case: If all else fails, if communication begins to break down, focus on the decision—how your problem will be treated. History, exam, and assessment are vital, but the decision is paramount. Always be sure that you are actively involved in any decision your doctor or HMO makes.

What Can I Do with Dr. Difficult?

In the days before managed care, the answer to this question was simple: go elsewhere. There was always another doctor ready to extend a helping hand. All it took was a phone call. These days, many patients have no choice. If you are in a staff or group model, for example, you might not even know whom you are going to see when you walk into your HMO. Those who get to choose a provider off a list might get a chance to change doctors if things don't work out, but often can only do so once a year. Managed care policy forces us to work with what we have.

This doesn't have to be a terrible thing. Continuity between a doctor and patient, even when it's forced as it might be in a PPO or IPA, has obvious benefits. The doctor knows the patient's history, remembers past treatments he prescribed, becomes familiar with the patient's personality, and can anticipate problems down the road. Doctors in a staff or group model rarely have this continuity, but when a patient makes an effort to work with them, rather than question them, it can brighten an otherwise routine day. This goes double for difficult doctors. When you bring them back from their preoccupations, assumptions, or role-playing, you have demonstrated a commitment that they don't often see.

You may not have this continuity if you are in a staff or group model, but in return you do have a built-in second opinion. If you see a different doctor each time, each will have the chance to check what their colleagues have done. As an informed and active patient, you can make up for the lack of continuity. Either way, you can turn the dictates of your HMO into a benefit.

There are many types of difficult doctors. Here, we are going to show you four. If you remember the four types of doctor-patient relationships from the second chapter, you can make a mutual relationship with your doctor a goal. Sometimes this means you need to empower your doctor, sometimes this means you need to empower yourself.

Dealing with Dr. Knowsbest

This is a doctor who prefers to have a paternalistic-type relationship with his patients. He is often condescending, dictating rather than negotiating a treatment plan. He prefers patients who feel they don't have much control in the examining room. He is the type of doctor who might not give you all the information you need—he assumes that you might not want to hear bad news, and you wouldn't understand anyway. When it comes to a diagnosis, he is rigid in his thinking. He knows he is right. He doesn't understand that a diagnosis is a *working diagnosis,* something that needs to be tested and questioned.

When you use HEAD with this type of doctor, you might not get the best results. He might not pay attention to your associated symptoms. He might focus on his first impression of the problem, and take control of the history, guiding it always to that first impression. He's a doctor with tunnel vision. The only thing he sees is his diagnosis. He isn't looking at the whole patient.

One of Dr. Theodosakis's encounters with this type of doctor turned tragic. A friend of his, "Gloria," had taken a vacation after separating from her husband. She suffered a forty-five-minute seizure and was taken to a local hospital. Her doctor gave her a brief examination and concluded that her seizure was a reaction to her recent breakup. His treatment plan was to get her into psychiatric care.

Gloria's relatives called Dr. Theodosakis and asked him to follow up with her doctor to make sure she was getting the best treatment. Dr. Theodosakis knew that the seizure *could* be caused by her emotional problems, but he also knew it could be more serious. When he talked to Gloria on the phone, he noticed her speech was slurred—a sign of meningitis. She reported seeing spots and colors, another sign. Dr. Theodosakis took the next step by asking her to touch her chin to her chest. "Oh, it hurts when I do that," she said. "I can't do it." Dr. Theodosakis knew that if Gloria had meningitis she could die if it wasn't treated. Testing was imperative.

But when Dr. Theodosakis got on the phone with Gloria's doctor, he hit a brick wall. The doctor's self-assured attitude came through even while talking to another doctor. "A spinal tap just isn't worth it in a case like this," he said. The message Dr. Theodosakis heard, however, was "Who are you to question my judgment?" The conversation rapidly turned ugly, with the belligerent doctor absolutely refusing to allow the test.

Dr. Theodosakis urged Gloria's family and friends to insist on the test, or to go elsewhere if they still couldn't get it. The doctor finally came around four days later, but by that time the disease had progressed too far to treat. In a month, she was dead from meningitis.

Doctors, like everyone else, make mistakes. But since doctors' mistakes put lives in danger, we rely on the checks and balances in HEAD to force us to question our own judgment. When you learn HEAD, you will have the power to ask those same questions. There isn't any problem with a doctor who forms first impressions. Gloria's doctor saw a young, recently separated woman who was under a great deal of emotional distress. That was one possible explanation for her seizure. But did it explain everything she was experiencing? Why was her speech slurred? Why was she seeing spots? Why did her neck hurt? Gloria's doctor failed to ask himself a fundamental and critical question: Does this diagnosis really make sense?

When your doctor explains your diagnosis, it should make sense. Just because you didn't go to medical school doesn't mean that you can't understand. Don't let your doctor tell you that this is beyond your understanding. It's all about you, and you have a need to know.

Using HEAD with Dr. Knowsbest will require all your powers of diplomacy. You want to show him that while you are empowered in the examining room, you are not taking any power away from him. Saying something like "I think this might be meningitis" probably won't work. He thinks he knows better than you. Showing Dr. Knowsbest articles you have found about your condition probably won't work for the same reason.

Instead, ask leading questions. Get back to your associated symptoms. Let him know how they affect you, how your life is changed by this condition. "I'm still worried about this pain in my side. What could that be?" Give him every opportunity to rethink his original assumption. "Could this develop into something more serious? Could it be something more serious?" Remember that this doctor is wearing blinders. Work to help him take them off. If he can't or won't, get a new doctor.

Dealing with Dr. Interruption

Most patients don't know what you know about how to give a history. That means that most doctors are ready to interrupt you in midsentence to get to the heart of the matter quickly. One study found that doctors interrupt their patients' response to their opening questions within fifteen seconds 69 percent of the time. Patients who were allowed to continue uninterrupted answered the opening question in an average of two and a half minutes. That's far too long for one question. If you're in a ten-minute visit, there's no way you can take this much time to answer the opening question: "What seems to be the problem?" It's no wonder that doctors feel the need to interrupt.

If you stick to HEAD, your doctor won't have such a pressing need to cut you off. But some doctors will be so used to taking control of the history that they can't help it. Some doctors will see a possible source of the problem right away, and will drive the history toward testing their assumption. Dr. Interruption is a doctor who is used to having control. But that doesn't mean that you can't share control during the visit.

If you are going through the steps in HEAD and your doctor starts asking questions that don't follow the format, let her. You should be thinking about where in HEAD she has jumped to or returned to. That will allow you to give organized information when you answer her questions. A doctor doesn't interrupt just because she thinks she knows best, so don't take an interruption as an insult. She could be interrupting because she sees something that inspires her to move toward a conclusion. She could be interrupting because you've left something out. She could be guiding you to a cure.

Read your doctor. Pay attention to her body language and tone. If she isn't being defensive when you start using HEAD, but interrupts anyway, you are probably in good hands. But don't stop paying attention. Remember where you were when the interruption came. Return to that point if you feel it is important. Make sure that you brought up everything on your list. Make sure that the interruption doesn't take your relationship with your doctor from mutuality to paternalism.

Dealing with Dr. Burnout

Dr. Burnout is a product of his managed care environment. He sees dozens of patients a day, he's seen his compensation cut, and he sees no end in sight. Unlike Dr. Knowsbest and Dr. Interruption, this doctor is in a position of low power. He questions his own judgment almost to the point of paralysis, and then he knows that the HMO will turn around and question it again. His patients are beginning to all look the same, and his utilization review doctor snuffs out any innovative spark that might inspire his suggestions for their treatment. He hears his patients without listening to them, and avoids getting his hands dirty with a physical exam. To get anything but cursory care from Dr. Burnout, you will have to find a way to empower him and inspire him.

Whatever else you do, don't approach this doctor like a consumer. Don't make him feel cornered by you on the one side and the HMO on the other. If you remember the four types of relationships from the second chapter, you can place Dr. Burnout in the "low doctor control" column. Either he will have a stagnant relationship with his patients, or his patients will act like consumers, questioning him at every turn and not following their prescribed treatment plans. You have been empowered by learning HEAD. Now you have a chance to share that power with your doctor.

Dr. Feinberg works too hard and gets excruciating migraine headaches about once a month. When he's in the grips of one of these headaches, he admits he's on the verge of burning out. He can't stand being at work, but rescheduling a day's worth of psychotherapy patients isn't possible. But when he is able to say something that actually helps his patient, when he really hits the nail on the head, the headache goes away. It's as if the ability to heal heals him.

If you have a doctor with a case of burnout, work on presenting your case as a problem to be solved. How can you make it interesting for your doctor? How can you make yourself stand out from the long line of patients waiting to see him? Try to tie your chief complaint to an associated symptom, life change, or piece of your social history. Would this give him a problem to solve?

Ask him about his past experience. "Have you seen this before?" He might start thinking about puzzle pieces he wouldn't have considered otherwise. He might remember a happier time before the coming of the HMOs, and might remember how he treated such problems back then.

Try letting him know when he has helped you. If you just walk out the door saying "Thanks," you are just another patient. Let him know that he has really helped. When he explains your problem, try giving him feedback. If it makes sense to you, tell him you understand. "That explains everything," "I get it," or "I totally see your point" will let him know that he has done a good job, and not just a job.

Were you referred to this doctor? Let him know, during the "source of referral" step of HEAD, how you came to him. If he came highly recommended, let him know. Have you been with this doctor for a long time and noticed he's been slowly burning out? Let him know you are worried about him with a question like "Any vacation plans this year?" Let him know why you have stayed with him all these years.

Perhaps you don't have the time for personal niceties in the space of a ten-minute office visit. Perhaps your doctor doesn't seem receptive. In cases like these, bring your doctor gifts. Not expensive ones, but just something thoughtful. Even a card or a letter will do. Dr. Feinberg's wife, also a doctor, once received a jar of homemade pasta sauce from a patient she had treated for pneumonia. The patient, who she knew was poor, had wrapped up the jar in elaborate paper and ribbons. There's no chance she will ever forget this patient or give him a cursory exam.

Dealing with Dr. Rush

Here's another product of managed care. Doctors who rushed through a patient's visit just to get to the next one used to be frowned upon. Now everyone's in a hurry. Some doctors have adapted to the new pace; others still have a lot to learn. Mara's doctor, back in chapter 1, is an example of a doctor who has allowed time restrictions to interfere with his relationships with patients. Any doctor who actually ignores complaints is ignoring his duty.

By using HEAD, you have established a reasonable, manageable pace for getting through the history and exam. Most doctors will immediately be put at ease, confident they can get everything done in ten minutes, or even become so fascinated with the problem you have presented that they will disregard the time restrictions. But some doctors won't slow down. They're used to asking one or two questions, taking a few quick notes, and sending the patient packing as soon as possible.

What they might not realize is that the HMO has diluted their power. Patients won't trust them, listen to them, or follow their treatment programs. Without gathering the information they need, they don't really have the power to make decisions. So the best tactic to dealing with a rushed doctor isn't to confront him, but to empower him with information.

Make eye contact. If Dr. Rush asks you what the problem is, but keeps looking through her charts or mail, don't answer until she looks at you. Once you have eye contact, move through HEAD in a way that lets the doctor know you are time-sensitive. Get right to the problem, get through the history, and when it comes time to plan, try to keep her there, focused on you. Saying things like "I just need a minute of your time. I have a few more questions about this treatment," or "This really has me concerned, can you explain further," should slow down a rushed doctor.

Since you are already using HEAD and doing everything you can to help streamline the visit, there's really no excuse for the doctor to feel rushed. But don't let that fact lead to a confrontation. If you fight with your doctor, there's little chance you will get more care than you have before. You can prod, but doing so subtly and politely will always get you further.

Recognizing Dr. Hopeless: Some Warning Signs

By now you will have realized that we believe you should work with your doctor. Most doctors are compassionate, caring, and intelligent people. Even the difficult cases carry deep within the original spark that sent them to medical school. If you can pull that out, you will get the care you deserve, HMO or no HMO. Having said that, there are times when you should change doctors.

We are in an incredibly stressful profession. Doctors suffer inordinately from mental illness, substance abuse, and suicide. The potential to make money at the expense of patients' health is ever present. The power doctors hold, we are sorry to say, makes some of them think they are above reproach. There are a number of warning signs you should be aware of and watch out for.

- Refusal to admit mistakes—This is a tough thing for doctors to do. We are supposed to be infallible. However, large and small mistakes do happen. Doctors fear that lawsuits tend to follow the admission of mistakes, but studies show patients are less likely to sue for malpractice if the doctor is forthright. A doctor who won't admit a mistake could be endangering your life. There's obviously something more important to him than your health. Move on.

- Inattentiveness to complaints—Always report your complaints. If they aren't addressed, keep reporting them in the way we showed you in the previous chapter. If your doctor refuses to look into why you are experiencing a problem, he has a problem. Even worse are doctors who say things like "You couldn't possibly have those symptoms." Outrageous statements like these are just attempts to get you to quit complaining. Go find someone who cares.

- Refusal to explain diagnoses—The first time you hear your diagnosis, you might not understand. You will want to ask questions until you do understand. Most doctors will work with you toward this goal. But we have also heard about doctors who just won't explain how they arrive at their conclusions, who make statements along the lines of "It's a flu because I say it's a flu." A doctor is not like an umpire. He can't just call them like he sees them. He has to have reasons. If your doctor tries to explain, try to understand. If your doctor *refuses* to explain, it's time to switch.

- Rigid thinking—Medical school training teaches doctors to be flexible, but a few get through without acquiring this important skill. The doctor who treated Dr. Theodosakis's friend Gloria was so rigid in his thinking that he couldn't see the warning signs of meningitis before him. All doctors should know that if the patient's signs and symptoms don't follow the expected course of the disease, there might be something wrong with the diagnosis. If your doctor won't change his diagnosis or plan, there's something wrong with your doctor.

- Refusal to conduct proper exam—Your doctor has to touch you. Taking subjective information (the history) isn't enough. Your doctor also needs objective information before he can know what to do. Sometimes the process can be as simple as taking your temperature or looking down your throat, but he has to examine you. If your doctor won't do this, even after you have invited him to look at or touch the problem area, you should examine your relationship with your doctor.

- Ethical transgressions—If your bill is consistently wrong, if your doctor tells you to forget about your Medicare co-payment, he's breaking the law. Even if this doesn't affect you, or works out in your favor, it's a telling sign. If he's willing to cross this line, how far will he go? When will your health be jeopardized for the sake of a few dollars?

- Sexual advances—There's no question here. If your doctor makes sexual advances toward you, he has violated the trust that underpins your relationship with him. If anything he does even seems inappropriate, don't wait for it to get worse. It's time to go.

The problems we have just mentioned are unlikely to come up. Most doctors are struggling with their HMOs, just like you are. Most will be ready to work with you once they see that you are an organized, committed patient. Perhaps one out of ten will need a little extra work before he is ready for a mutual relationship. Perhaps one out of a hundred will be a hopeless case. We've tried to give you additional tools to use with these tough cases, and warning signs that will tell you when to give up. Next we'd like to concentrate on problems that originate with patients, and show how you can HEAD these off.

How Does HEAD Make Me a "Good" Patient?

When some doctors call a patient "good," they are sometimes referring to how good their insurance is. But when you bring HEAD into the examining room, you can become a good patient even without "good" insurance. You've elevated yourself from passive patient to active participant, a move almost any doctor will appreciate.

Now, however, we should give you a few words of warning about the method you have just learned. HEAD doesn't make you a doctor. It makes you a near-perfect patient, but your doctor is still the one who will diagnose your problem and initiate the treatment. By entering your health maintenance organization armed with HEAD, you have shifted your role and your doctor's. Some of the problem doctors we mentioned above won't be quite ready for this, which is why we urge a persevering, diplomatic approach. Now it's time to prepare yourself for your new role as a mutual partner in your health care decisions.

Your doctor is not a god, magician, or father figure, and you should always avoid seeing him as such. This does not demean his position. He doesn't have to be cast up to Olympian heights in order to do his job. In today's medical world, with their every move ultimately governed by the HMOs, it's impossible to hold onto the image we used to have of our doctors. We are all coming around to the idea that health care is a business, and your doctor can fairly be viewed as a professional—a highly trained, well-educated, and deeply committed professional.

When you avoid seeing your doctor in the stereotypical role of miracle-worker, you open up new lines of communication. The doctor doesn't have to live up to an expectation that's beyond him. He can get back to genuine behavior, he can be himself, and he can be spontaneous, even within the restrictions of the HMO.

At the same time, your role is also changing. You aren't the old-fashioned patient who blindly followed the doctor's lead. You won't restrict yourself to giving the doctor only the information he directly asks for. You won't act until you are sure you understand. But at the same time, you aren't just a consumer. You approach the doctor from a position of trust, rather than suspicion. You know to use HEAD as a tool for communication, not for interrogation.

Now that you have gained new understanding of how your doctor thinks about you and your condition, it is more important than ever for you to understand your role as a patient. A little knowledge can be a dangerous thing, especially when you are using it in front of someone who really knows what she's talking about. Make sure that you use HEAD to ask questions of yourself and your doctor. Never use it to jump to conclusions.

An elderly man we knew walked into his HMO emergency room one day with a bad cough that he'd had for three days. When the doctor he saw asked what was wrong, he replied, "I think it might be pneumonia." The doctor shot back: "That's a diagnosis, not your symptoms." The doctor reached for some over-the-counter cough medicine and tried to move him along. The patient became very worried and asked if the cough medicine was sufficient. He asked if the doctor could take a closer look. Begrudgingly, the doctor took his temperature, and was immediately relieved that he had—the patient had a temperature of 103. The patient went home with antibiotics to treat his pneumonia.

What went wrong here? Both the doctor and the patient made mistakes; both were lucky that they questioned the situation further. But all the bad feelings between them could have been avoided if they had started off on the right foot. Rather than answering the doctor's question, the patient jumped to a conclusion. It happened to be the correct one, but it was still not what the doctor wanted to hear. Moving straight to a diagnosis goes against his medical training. It's almost insulting for a patient to skip the steps that he's spent years learning. The lesson we can learn from this nearly tragic situation is that a guess can be dangerous to your health, whether it's your guess or your doctor's.

If you have an idea of what you might have, explain first your reasons for thinking so. Give a complete history. The patient in the example above focused only on his cough, failing to mention his fever. The patient didn't answer the doctor's question, which only made the doctor think he was a difficult patient.

We are not trying to blame the victim in this case. The doctor failed in his duty to look at the patient, and that was wrong. If the patient had gone home with cough medicine instead of antibiotics, his fate would have been on the doctor's shoulders. But the point of the story isn't to assign blame. We only want you to think about how your words and actions might aggravate an overworked, underpaid, underappreciated physician.

Being an active patient does not mean you should play doctor. You still need your doctor's honest opinion and you still need to let him know that you respect the role he plays in your health. You might have to show some humility. You might have to swallow a little pride. Don't let that bother you. If you use HEAD to communicate, you will earn back the small sacrifice of pride a thousand times over.

What Else Do I Need to Know about Treatment Plans?

The best feeling you can have as a patient is walking out the door knowing what's wrong with you, knowing what you can do about it, and knowing that you have been cared for. It's the moment that makes both doctor and patient cherish their relationship. To get there you must stay involved in the discussion of your treatment plan; you want the mutuality of your relationship to shine through.

Studies of doctors' and patients' decision making show some disturbing trends, but also show the way toward hope. Doctors are learning through these surveys that patients are generally not satisfied with their consultations, something patients rarely tell them face-to-face. Doctors are also learning what they can do about this general lack of satisfaction. The most common reason patients give for their discontent is that they were not able to describe their own goals during the course of the visit. A doctor might be able to make you well, but what you really want is information on how to not get sick in the first place.

Dissatisfaction with the consultation goes beyond just the feeling of being left out. A good consultation has a very real therapeutic effect that precedes and promotes whatever treatment program is ultimately decided upon. Studies of chronic patients suggest that those who take part in the decision-making process improve their situation more often than those who don't. These patients take their medicine consistently, avoid damaging behaviors, and really work to change their lifestyles. Patients who aren't active in the decision-making process typically fail to do any of these things. In fact, only about a third of all patients follow their treatment plan exactly the way their doctor ordered. This is a real and serious health problem, but we know the cure. Let the patient into the decision-making process. Let him make decisions himself. Empower the patient and he will be motivated to cure himself.

Following the treatment plan as an empowered patient means more than just taking the pills. You should be aware of the course that your problem is expected to take. How soon will it get better? What should you watch out for along the way?

An HMO patient who later became a patient of Dr. Theodosakis injured his shoulder while playing baseball. He asked to see an

---

CREATING A TREATMENT PLAN: TIPS FOR ACTIVE PATIENTS

- Allow as much time as possible. You will need at least two minutes. Try to get more.

- Match your doctor's explanations to your symptoms. Be sure you understand how your symptoms are related to his diagnosis.

- Use "we" as often as possible: What are we going to do next? When will we know if this decision is right?

- State your goals. What do you really want out of this treatment? Try to expand your goal beyond this particular illness.

- When you have to reevaluate a treatment plan, ask what went wrong. Think about what you might have left out of the history, or what symptoms the doctor might have left out of his decision.

- Once the plan is established, be sure to find out how far your plan will cover the treatment. How much medicine can you take before coverage runs out? How many physical therapy visits are covered? If this plan doesn't work, where does that leave me?

orthopedic surgeon, but his plan guided him to his primary care physician first. Unfortunately, he was told he had to suffer a two-week wait before his PCP could squeeze him in. By the time his PCP looked at his shoulder, he was angry and acted curt and dismissive with the doctor. All he wanted out of the visit was a referral to an orthopedic surgeon. This kept him from giving a full history. He thought his words would be wasted on a nonspecialist.

The primary care physician didn't have all the information he needed to do his job properly. The result was a diagnosis of "rotator cuff tear." The prescription: physical therapy. By now the patient was even angrier, but assumed the role of the dutiful patient and followed the doctor's routine. The shoulder pain got worse during physical therapy, but the patient didn't know what to think of the pain. Was it just part of the course of getting better? Or was it a warning sign that the diagnosis was wrong? The patient endured the increasing pain for weeks before it became unbearable and he finally returned to his PCP. He was then allowed to see an orthopedic surgeon.

The specialist wasted no time getting to the root of the problem. The patient had been aggravating a fractured humerus during physical therapy. Now surgery was required. The surgery went well, but the patient needed additional physical therapy to treat his now-repaired shoulder. Since he had been in physical therapy for weeks already, however, his entire allotment of visits was used up and the HMO refused to pay. The patient developed a frozen shoulder and was out of work for more than a year.

HOW CAN I AVOID BEING HELPLESS IN THE HOSPITAL?

If you are ever admitted to the hospital, you will need all your team-building skills to make sure that you come out safely. Hospitals are not nice places to be. In addition to the risks associated with the procedures you will undergo, you are at risk every time you eat, get an injection, or take a drug. Team-building becomes more difficult when so many of the people treating you seem to come and go at random times. Now more than ever, it's important to stay focused and alert. Here are a few tips to get you safely to your discharge.

- If you are incapacitated, or don't feel you can be very assertive, bring someone you trust to advocate for you. Let them know exactly what you want them to watch out for.

HOW CAN I AVOID BEING HELPLESS (continued)

- Find out before you go what the plan for discharging you is. How will they know it's okay to let you go? What complications might prevent the planned discharge?

- Get your nurse practitioner on your side. Besides being a medical professional, she also knows about social work issues like getting counseling for your family, arranging transportation, even hooking you up with someone who can feed your dog.

- Nurses sometimes come through quickly to execute instructions from your doctor. If those instructions involve giving you an IV, injection, or drugs, be absolutely sure to ask what they are doing before it goes into your body. A simple question will make them think twice, and may allow them to catch a mistake before it happens.

- If a nurse is having trouble inserting a needle or IV, don't suffer in silence. Give them two or three chances, and then ask for a break. They may then go find someone who's an expert at finding veins.

- Notify your nurse if the injection point develops any swelling, redness, or itching. The needle may be poorly inserted, and the process may have to be done over.

- If you have a strong fear of needles, say so. This will allow the nurse to take extra precautions.

- If you are in the hospital for surgery, be sure to talk to your anesthesiologist before your operation. Give a complete history to the anesthesiologist, paying special attention to your social and family history. If anyone in your family has experienced malignant hyperthermia, you could have a deadly reaction to anesthesia. Also be sure to tell her about dentures and other mouth appliances. Find out what she's going to do, what the dangers are, and what your options are. Make sure she sees you as a person.

- You will be seeing all sorts of people, with very different jobs. Find out from each person who treats you who they are and what their title is. Just don't make them feel defensive about it.

- Don't leave if you are in doubt about your condition. Signs like fever, confusion, disorientation, inability to take fluids orally, or faintness should make you or your advocate question a discharge. Ask about the appeals process, write a note by hand, and have a friend or family member deliver it immediately.

- On the other hand, you should get out of there as soon as you are out of danger. At home you can get more rest, there's less risk of an infection, and you will be much happier. Learning things like how to change your own dressing or coordinating a caregiver can help the process along.

What went wrong here? First, the patient didn't give a full history. He expected to be referred to a specialist. Remember that you will never have your expectations met in a managed care environment if you don't give a full history. Doctors in HMOs aren't encouraged to go looking for problems. You have to present them. Second, the patient stuck with a treatment plan that wasn't working. If he had understood the plan, he would have known that the increasing pain was a warning sign. If he had been an active participant in reaching the treatment decision, he might have raised objections to physical therapy: "I don't know if I can do that. The pain is far too bad." He could have given the doctor a chance to reconsider his mistaken diagnosis and reach the correct one.

The real tragedy of this case lies in the fact that the patient used up his allotted visits, making his problem worse. Always remember that in managed care, you often only have one or two chances to get well before you are cut off. This harsh reality means that it's even more important for you to be aware of your body and how your treatment plan is affecting it. You can never assume that you will get another chance to correct your doctor's mistake. Never be afraid to tell him if his treatment plan isn't working.

What Have I Accomplished?

Using HEAD can do more than get you through the ten-minute exam. It can calm difficult doctors, and inspire burned-out doctors. But even outside the examining room, HEAD keeps working. If you can use this method of cataloging your health history, you will begin to see where your general health can improve. You can start to define goals for the maintenance of your own health. The next chapter will concentrate on how you can use clues in your medical history to define preventive treatment goals. Using the information you've gathered through HEAD, in conjunction with your HMO's resources, you will learn how to keep yourself healthy and out of the examining room as much as possible.

~ 5 ~

Preventive Medicine

The High Road to Health

QUESTIONS THIS CHAPTER ANSWERS

◆ *Why should I care about prevention?*

◆ *How do I prepare for healthful change?*

◆ *How do I pick a diet?*

◆ *How do I pick my dietary supplements?*

◆ *How can I establish an exercise program?*

◆ *How can sleep, environment, and social interactions keep me healthy?*

◆ *How can my HMO help?*

Your HMO can't kill you if you don't get sick. If you have good health, maintain it, and stay on top of a schedule of screenings, you can be your own health maintenance organization, a savvy customer who keeps health insurance ready for serious problems and regular check-ups.

The open secret of the medical profession is that almost all of the premature deaths by disease in this country could have been prevented by lifestyle changes. Why we (and our doctors) ignore this fact is a mystery. Although most preventive measures leave your HMO on the sidelines, we knew we couldn't write a book called *Don't Let Your HMO Kill You* without giving you a few prevention tips that can save your life.

Dr. Theodosakis started out in internal medicine, training to become a specialist in adult care. As his medical career progressed, he reached the conclusion that treating disease after it happened was not enough. He too often felt like he was standing on the bank of a fast-flowing river, waiting to pluck out patients who had fallen in and were being swept helplessly downstream. After being forced to rescue some of the same patients more than once, he decided to try to get to the patients *before* they fell in, *prevent* their disease before it started. It made sense to him, and probably makes sense to you, but your managed care company probably hasn't figured out that preventing disease is the simplest and best way to keep their members healthy.

Preventive medicine is recognized by the medical establishment, but most managed care companies leave it out of their programs. It's the most effective and cheapest strategy for health care, but the managed care companies don't seem all that interested. Why should that be the case? The answer, like so many answers to managed care questions, has to do with the almighty dollar.

There's always the chance that a positive screening test may result in huge outlays on further testing or treatment. A patient may come into the office with no symptoms, get an HIV test, and a few days later, if the test is positive, the HMO may have to start paying for treatments that cost over $1,000 per month.

In the strictest business terms, the company is likely to save money by not providing the screening test at all. The patient might walk around for years with asymptomatic HIV, while the plan saves $1,000 for each month the diagnosis is delayed. However disturbing it may be, we have to understand the way some plan managers think: that the plan saves money if the patient dies of AIDS soon after being diagnosed rather than requiring months or years of life-sustaining treatment. It's not such a big leap from thinking that way to actively creating roadblocks that prevent timely diagnosis.

Sound far-fetched? It really isn't. This practice happens on a daily basis. In 1996, data from the National Committee for Quality Assurance (NCQA) revealed huge differences between the best plans and the worst plans regarding routine screening for several diseases for which early diagnosis is key to survival. The managed care plans with the worst records screened only 25 percent of eligible members for cervical cancer, 10 percent for diabetes, 30 percent for breast cancer, and 15 percent for heart disease—a sad picture indeed.

Fortunately, pressure from patients, employers, patient advocate groups, "insider" prevention advocates, and government regulators is forcing the managed care industry into offering some preventive services. You may need to apply pressure yourself, but first you need to know what to ask for. We will discuss the issue of screenings later in the chapter, and give you an accessible list of disease-specific interventions in appendix C. But first, we would like to share with you the key to prevention—behavior change—and give you some specific tips on the preventive measures that start at home.

How Can I Prepare for Healthful Change?

The worst part of those long stays in the waiting room is the way your mind can wander. You just know it's going to be cancer, after all, you can feel the lump. You start to wallow in regret: "Why didn't I quit smoking earlier? Why did I allow myself to gain so much weight? How could I let myself skip my mammogram *two years in a row?*" You promise yourself and God that if things turn out well, that if you survive, you'll lead a totally different lifestyle and do all of the things you know are good for you.

The second-worst part of being a doctor is telling a patient they are going to die. So what's the worst part of the job? Seeing a person weeping from regret over the things they "should have done." The patient knows he's helpless to stop the course of a disease, but he also knows that at some point in the past he could have made the right choices. When he learns that his death is imminent, all he can do is wonder, How could I have been so stupid?

Change isn't easy, especially when it involves changing bad habits. Even when we know we should change it's always easier to stay the same. It's hardly ever a lack of information that allows unhealthy behaviors to continue. The obstacles are usually emotional.

The underlying issue often begins with a sort of "emotional disconnection" that helps perpetuate the resistance to change. For example, a person who thinks little of himself will find it very difficult to care enough to change. Why? Because unconsciously he doesn't feel he's worth it. This problem involves a conflict between the conscious decision to take care of oneself and the unconscious belief that one is destined to be a failure. What one *really* believes about oneself has far more power than what one *wants* to believe.

Successful change requires transforming old beliefs into new possibilities. We must understand our emotions and recognize how we think and talk to ourselves. Finally, change requires a realistic vision of possibilities and a concrete set of goals.

It's always best to take baby steps when making changes, as radical change can often lead to anxiety and fear. However, there is no greater motivator than the power you obtain from your own actions. Let's take a look at how this was demonstrated by one of Dr. Theodosakis's patients.

When Wendy turned eleven years old she went on her first diet. Teased both at school and at home about her weight, she would virtually starve herself for days. Finally, Wendy lost a lot of weight and temporarily gained the praise she had been seeking. Later that year, however, she gained it all back and was more depressed than ever. Now, at forty-six, she recalls repeating this cycle dozens of times, losing weight then gaining it back. Sometimes she'd gain more than she lost.

Wendy described feeling hopeless and confused. She tearfully admitted she was afraid to give it another try. She just couldn't understand why all of her nutrition and exercise knowledge had failed her. "What am I missing, Doc?" she would ask. "You keep trying to fix what isn't broken," Dr. Theodosakis told her. "Knowledge isn't your problem, fear is your problem." It was at that point that Wendy was ready to begin to piece together her history of self-sabotage with her true feelings about her body. For years her greatest obstacle had been her fear of failure, rejection, and ridicule.

When you are unable to consciously identify the true nature of the problem, the tendency is to return to old behaviors. While this response is obviously irrational, many people continue to fall victim to this pattern. To succeed, it's essential to understand the underlying reasons you are sabotaging your own efforts. This is the first step toward long-term change.

While you are exploring the true nature of your resistance, it's important to initiate the active change process as well. Your bad habits will disappear when you experience yourself trying new things, challenging yourself in new ways, and changing your self-image.

For instance, you may start to view yourself as more athletic after you notice the improvements in your muscle tone and stamina with just a few weeks of regular exercise. Other people in your life may notice the change, and reinforce your new feelings about yourself. The encouragement from those around you will contribute to your success by supporting the behaviors that reflect your true self.

Counseling and therapy are wonderful ways to knock down emotional obstacles, but they become nothing more than "psychobabble" if you're not actively taking steps to do things differently. Wendy went to psychotherapy to help her understand just how her past had negatively influenced her behavior. While attending weekly therapy, she also joined a health club and hired a personal trainer. Wendy had tried this in the past, but this time she was working on shedding emotional baggage at the same time she was shedding pounds.

For the first time Wendy knew what she wanted and how to get there. She made sure that her exercises were enjoyable and fun. She refused to force herself into activities that were too difficult or tedious. For emotional exercise, Wendy began each day with a ten-minute visual meditation on the woman she longed to be. While negative thoughts would still come knocking, she now had the strength to send them away. She said to Dr. Theodosakis, laughing, "You know, Doc, when those old thoughts come into my head I just say to myself, 'Thank you for sharing, now GET OUT!'"

As Wendy's body changed and strengthened, so did her opinion of herself. She had taken ownership of her body and mind, guaranteeing that both would be permanently transformed.

Personal change is an art. It takes vision, technique, and commitment—things we can all possess. Here are a few steps that will help you to discover and maintain your new vision of yourself as you practice the art of change.

- Remember that you're not just looking for new things to do. You are looking for new behaviors that create *new ways to feel*.

- Begin each day with deep breathing and a short visualization of your vision for change. Before you get out of bed in the morning, take five to ten minutes to close your eyes and envision yourself as the person you know you can be. Visualizing is both relaxing and extremely powerful in terms of bringing you back to your initial feelings about wanting to take permanent control of your habits.

- Each day, write down the specific changes you are going to make for that day. Put the list in a place where you often look, such as the bathroom mirror or the pantry door. Be specific with your targets.

- Identify your obstacles by writing them down one at a time. Then, list three solutions for each obstacle. For example, let's say one obstacle

is your resistance to exercise. One solution could be finding exercises
you enjoy, such as dancing. Another could be setting time aside to
dance in the morning, and a third could be a reward, like purchasing
new music every two weeks.

- Actively participate in behavior that supports your vision. This is the
  most important part because no one can truly change unless they
  actually experience themselves differently in the change process.
  Take note of your physical changes and how they create an emotional
  change. Watch how your emotional changes allow you to take physical action. It's a beautiful process, once you see how it works.

Nothing can take away the emotional high you receive from getting past your fears and knowing that you and only you made it possible. Eventually, the things you should be doing will become a part of
who you really are. A simple but poignant example is brushing your
teeth. You probably hated brushing your teeth as a child—most kids
do. With constant, often willful repetition—often urged, of course, by
your parents—you eventually incorporated brushing your teeth into
your daily routine. Now it's so much a part of you that you would
probably feel terrible if someone kept you from brushing. This same
type of "automatic incorporation" into your everyday life can occur
with almost any healthy behavior.

Another important step is gathering support from others who will
believe in you. Reinforce your success by spending time with people
who have similar goals. Knowing you're not alone is both comforting
and healing. You can be both a receiver and giver of strength, knowledge, and hope. Self-help books are fine, but they can't replace the
warmth and strength you get from good friends or people going
through similar struggles.

Finally, be warm to yourself. Speak kindly to yourself. Nothing
destroys hope faster than negative self-talk. Unkind thoughts can
quickly spiral into hopelessness. Consider keeping a journal of your
thoughts and feelings and observe just how often you beat yourself
up. Practicing positive thoughts will create the hope and courage you
need to actively seek the changes you've longed for.

The principles of behavior change are the foundation for good preventive health, and they will work for any type of change, from quit-
ting smoking to remembering to take your vitamins. These are things
that you have to do on your own—most HMOs won't even help you

quit smoking, even though it's clear that they would save money by doing so. In fact, the rise of managed care means that we have to take a bigger role in managing our own health.

How Can I Change My Diet?

"Eat right." We've heard these words from the time we were children. It's hard enough to do when junk food and snacks tempt us at every turn, but on top of that, we get all sorts of mixed messages about what "eating right" really means.

More than half of us admit in surveys that we feel confused about diet and supplement information. One day eggs are evil, the next day a new study finds that people who eat eggs aren't any less healthy than those who don't. One published doctor says we should stay away from carbohydrates, another says we should stay away from proteins. Who's right?

There's only thing anyone can say for certain about diets: *There is no one healthy diet that works for everyone.* When you are choosing a diet you have to pay attention to your individual needs. For example:

- Your medical condition—Certain medical conditions require special diets. People with high cholesterol and coronary artery disease require a lower-fat diet and people with adult-onset diabetes require diets with fewer simple sugars.

- Your stage of life—People's dietary needs change throughout their lives. This is especially evident with older people who have a decreased ability to absorb certain nutrients such as Vitamin B_{12} and calcium.

- Your ethnic background—It's amazing how different we are regarding our ability to process certain foods. Even people who look the same on the outside can be very different on the inside. For example, some people's ancestors lived in regions where there was very little iron in the soil, and therefore little iron in their foods. They evolved an ability to absorb more iron from their diet, which was a benefit for them, but a potential problem for their descendants. About one in two hundred people have this trait: when eating a typical iron-rich American diet, iron is deposited in excessive amounts throughout their bodies. They can develop heart disease, diabetes, and liver problems as a result.

These are just a few of the reasons why there's no such thing as a "one size fits all" diet. As you develop a diet plan, be sure to consult your doctor or nutritionist, take into account your special health needs, and above all, pay attention to your own body's reactions to food and stick with what makes you feel healthy. Even though your diet will follow your individual needs, there are a few pieces of general advice that have stood the test of time, and apply to most everyone:

Eat a Wide Variety of Fruits and Vegetables

The "five a day" slogan is a good start, but really seven to nine per day for most people would be better. A wide variety of fruits and vegetables assures that you'll get a wide variety of nutrients, some of which have not even been discovered. Diets high in fruits and vegetables have shown clinical improvement in many diseases, including inflammatory arthritis (such as rheumatoid arthritis), diabetes, and heart disease. In addition, the lowest rates of many types of cancers are found in those people who have higher vegetable and fruit intake. Vegetables appear to be more protective than fruit. Not everyone feels great on a strict vegetarian diet, so the addition of fish and low-fat turkey, chicken, or other high-protein foods is advisable for some. But although a varied vegetarian diet can be one of the healthiest, strict vegan diets (which allow no animal products) are often deficient in vitamins B_2, B_3, B_{12}, calcium, and iron, so supplements may be needed.

Expand Your Rotation of Meals

Most families eat the same eight to ten dishes at home because this is generally the limit of the cook's repertoire. Even if all the foods included are vitamin-rich and low-fat, this diet will inevitably miss important nutrients. Try to add one new and healthy meal each month, and let this become a regular part of the rotation. Let the less healthy meals drop out of the rotation gradually, and your family won't even miss them. Improving eating patterns by addition of healthier choices is the best way to achieve a good diet in the long run. We too often hear about what foods to eliminate, but if there aren't good choices to replace the less healthy meals, you're likely to feel deprived and will quickly fall back on your old food choices.

Meal variety has another benefit, often not publicized. There are about one million naturally occurring chemicals found in foods. Some of these are cancer-promoting (carcinogenic) and are no less risky than synthetic chemicals, such as pesticides. The varied diet limits your risk from both natural and synthetic chemicals that can cause your body harm.

Eat Natural Fats and Steer Clear of Artificially Altered Fat

Ever wonder why some groups of people have relatively high-fat diets but have much lower rates of diseases such as clogged arteries and heart attacks? All fats are not created equal; some are in fact much better than others. The diet message in much of the 1980s and '90s— "fat is the enemy"—left out this important fact. It's become more and more clear that while the amount of fat in a diet is important, the *kind* of fat in a diet is even more important.

Fat is one of our four energy sources, carbohydrates, protein, and alcohol being the others. Fats (solid at room temperature) and oils (fats that are liquid at room temperature) are certain groups of molecules that contain a string of carbon atoms with attached hydrogen atoms. When each of the carbon atoms reaches its maximum of attached hydrogen atoms (three on the end carbon molecules and two on the middle ones), the fat is *saturated* or *hydrogenated*. If only one of the carbons is missing a hydrogen atom, the fat is *monounsaturated*. If there are several carbons without hydrogen, the fat is *polyunsaturated*. You've seen these terms before. Just look at the labels and ingredient lists on most processed foods in the store.

Animal fat tends to be saturated fat. It is solid at room temperature and causes health problems if eaten in large quantities. Vegetable oils span the fat spectrum. Almost all contain a mixture of the three types of fat. Palm kernel oil is high in saturated fat and low in the others. Olive oil is high in monounsaturated fats and low in the others. Olive oil and the fats in cold-water, deep-sea fish appear to be the best for your health.

Look at the labels on food products, but don't be fooled. Many food manufacturers use familiar and enticing phrases like "All natural," "100 percent vegetable oil," or " No cholesterol," but the fats in these products may be worse for you than raw pig lard! To make their products taste rich while using only vegetable oil, manufacturers use a process called hydrogenation. The result is a solid fat that won't drip out of the product and tastes like fully saturated animal fat; however, the process creates a by-product called *trans fat* that's just as dangerous, if not more dangerous, than animal fat. Your body isn't used to seeing trans fats in large quantities, but they make up over 20 percent of products such as stick margarine or shortening. Unfortunately, food labels are not required to list levels of trans fats. Trans fats are horrible for your health and may be the single biggest "no-no" in our diets. These fats reduce the body's production of high-density lipoprotein (HDL or "good cholesterol") and interfere with metabolism of normal fats. Gram for gram, they are actually riskier than saturated fats like animal fat, the kind we've long been told to avoid.

A study in the *New England Journal of Medicine* in November 1997 revealed that, among 80,000 nurses followed for up to fourteen years, those consuming the highest amount of trans fat had the highest heart attack rate. What was surprising to researchers was that it seemed to make little or no difference if the nurses' total fat consumption was a low or high percentage of their total calorie intake. This study is evidence that the *kind* of fat consumed is more important than the *quantity*. This helps explain why most bakery and fast-food products are killers. You can expect to learn soon that trans fat is related to cancer and other diseases much more than was previously believed.

What to do about your fats? Of course, stay away from fried foods, bakery products, and any food that lists hydrogenated or partially hydrogenated fats. You should consider using extra virgin olive oil as your mainstay. There's strong evidence for its benefits. Buy small bottles and keep them away from heat and light. We often pierce a few capsules of vitamin E to add to a newly opened bottle to help keep the oil from becoming rancid. Storing the bottle in the refrigerator is a good idea, but too often the fridge is too cold and the oil solidifies. There are some new margarine-like spreads on the market that claim to be devoid of trans fats. Whether or not they are healthier is anyone's guess at this time.

Watch the Alcohol

Newspapers and magazines love it when studies reveal that alcohol can be beneficial, but in truth alcohol is not healthy for most people.

These studies deal with populations, not individuals. Even the best testing to date can't establish if alcohol is safe for *anyone* to use on a long-term basis. Alcohol use affects your sleep quality, and is associated with several cancers, some of which are undetectable until they're advanced. Of course, people with osteoporosis, gout, liver problems such as hepatitis, people taking certain medications, and people with high blood pressure should consume very little, if any, alcohol.

Even putting aside these concerns, alcoholic beverages are full of calories, and that should be enough reason for most people to abstain. If you are a drinker, consider making a visit to your doctor to find out if there are any specific health reasons for you to avoid alcohol. You may be surprised by the results.

How Can I Control My Weight?

There's no magic formula for weight loss. Americans spend about $33 billion each year searching for one, but 98 percent of all interventions fail. Most dieters know that the solutions are in themselves, but they keep buying books and attending seminars that promise effortless solutions. Most of these programs are unproven fads, and it makes us sick to think that some of our colleagues are using their medical degrees to exploit Americans desperate to lose weight. They know that weight loss is a matter of behavioral change. Most dieters, deep down inside, know this as well. But we still search for the magic bullet, and there are plenty of quacks ready to say they've found it.

The National Weight Control Registry (NWCR) is one source worth listening to. The NWCR is a database of over 2,000 people, aged eighteen and over, who have lost at least thirty pounds and have kept it off for at least a year. By most definitions, this is successful weight loss. The average participant in the NWCR has lost about sixty pounds and kept it off for about five years. Two-thirds of these successful weight losers were overweight as children and 60 percent report that there's obesity in their families. They also report that they have made substantial changes in eating and exercise habits in order to lose weight and keep it off.

So what are some of the keys to long-term weight loss? How do people like the NWCR registrants, along with thousands of others, reach their goals? The answers are simple, but you don't often see them advertised or hyped in the media because no one can make money off them. You do these things at home, on your own, for little or no cost. Here are some of the "secrets."

- Eat low-fat diets—On average, the NWCR registrants reported consuming about 24 percent calories from fat. The average American consumes about 40–45 percent calories from fat. Despite the recent hype over high-fat, high-protein, and low-carbohydrate diets, low-fat diets are the ones that get long-term results.

- Exercise regularly—The average NWCR subject exercised off about four hundred calories per day. Most did this simply by walking. Some bought home equipment or joined a gym, especially if they wanted to lift weights, a highly recommended method of exercise for improving health and losing fat. An average-sized person can burn four hundred calories by walking for an hour. Keep in mind, without regular, almost daily exercise, there's virtually no hope of long-term weight control.

- Believe in yourself—About half of the success stories in the NWCR report losing weight totally on their own. No physician or group interventions, no "fat blockers," no chalky-tasting supplements, "diet" bars, or milkshakes.

- Do it for yourself—Most successful weight losers in the NWCR did it for themselves. They weren't just trying to look good for an upcoming wedding, class reunion, or beach vacation. Temporary goals yield temporary results.

- Set realistic goals—Genetic makeup has a lot to do with your upper and lower weight limits. Don't aspire to look like a skinny runway model if that's not your body type.

- Don't deprive yourself—Most NWCR participants didn't have to keep some foods completely "off-limits." There are foods that you can eat regularly and foods that you should limit. The important thing is to find a balance that works.

- Don't use drugs—Even herbal supplements, like the amphetamine-like substance ephedra, may be no healthier than prescription amphetamines. People who use drugs or herbs to maintain weight loss are sure to get it back if they stop using the drug. Some will even become addicted to the drug, and even more prone to health problems than if they had stayed overweight.

- Track your progress—That doesn't mean putting yourself on the scale. NWCR success stories track their exercise patterns, fitness levels, or levels of lean muscle. These are much better indicators than simple body weight.

- Stay organized and plan for the long term—Successful weight loss is created by simple choices with big effects. Staying at hotels with fitness centers, centering social activities around activity rather than food, or planning meals a week in advance are a few examples of NWCR "best practices." There may be some ups and downs, but that's normal. All humans, skinny and fat, have fluctuations in their weight. Despite these fluctuations, stick with the long-term game plan.

Weight loss and weight control is like a career. Suppose a high school or college counselor told his students there's only one thing they need to know for the future: "Go out and get a lot of money." Some particularly efficient kids might just go out and rob a bank. Of course, relying on such a get-rich-quick scheme tends to produce very unhappy consequences. The good counselor advises student to get an education, work hard, and stick with the program for the long haul. Graduates who are patient and diligent will end up establishing satisfying and challenging careers, and eventually be rewarded with financial security.

Advising people to "go on a diet" is just as unhelpful as telling them to get rich quick. The quick and fast weight loss schemes universally fail and leave their victims with false hope, further weight gain, lost income, and damage to self-esteem. Don't go "on a diet." Go out and change your life.

How Can Dietary Supplements Help?

Dietary supplements—vitamins, minerals, herbs, and "specialty products"—are a part of so many daily lives that we hardly think about them. About half of the U.S. population regularly take supplements, barely paying attention to the controversy that surrounds their use. Both critics and proponents of supplements seem just as fanatical about their positions, and both sides have plenty of good evidence.

Overall, the findings on supplement use are positive, but that doesn't necessarily mean they're right for you. It also doesn't mean your doctor will recommend them to you. Patients are frequently puzzled when their doctors won't recommend supplements, or even give advice on their use. Your doctor has plenty of good reasons, which we will go into next, but also plenty of reasons why they (and you) should be cautious.

Why Should I Take Supplements?

There are at least six main reasons why dietary supplements are needed for optimal health:

1. Not even the most disciplined person eats a healthy diet *all* of the time. All of us go through periods when we eat large amounts of foods we know we shouldn't, eat the same foods over and over (the so called "monotonous diet"), travel and forgo our routines, or miss out on fruits and vegetables, especially during the winter months. Whatever the cause for the deviation from the optimal diet, dietary supplements can help replace those nutrients that may be missing.

2. Supplements can "fill in" for lost nutrients that occur when food is processed. We'd love to recommend that you eat only fresh, unprocessed foods, but we know this is totally unpractical for most. No amount of supplementation can "fix" a diet based entirely on processed foods, but supplements can be a great benefit to those who combine fresh foods with processed foods.

3. Supplements can make up for varying levels of nutrients in foods. Fruits and vegetables grown on the same soil year after year can vary widely in levels of important nutrients. Two carrots grown at either end of the same field can be quite different in nutrient content. To complicate matters, crops harvested from depleted soil may be deficient in many nutrients, most notably trace minerals. There's no way to know if your broccoli, asparagus, or corn has a high or low level of selenium, for example.

4. Supplements can protect against toxins. Those of us who are deficient in minerals will find pesticides more toxic, for example. Lead poisoning is more acute for those who have calcium and iron deficiencies. These are just two examples out of many.

5. Some people can absorb nutrients more easily in supplement form. Older people, for example, have a diminished ability to digest and absorb many nutrients, even without the presence of a known disease. It is therefore possible to eat properly but still have some deficiencies if you can't absorb or utilize certain nutrients properly from food. The most common example is vitamin B_{12}. Our ability to

absorb B_{12} declines with age, even to the point where oral vitamin B_{12} supplements can be ineffective and the vitamin must be administered by injection.

6. Finally, and perhaps most important, it takes a high dose of nutrients to prevent or treat disease. Treating and preventing disease often requires people to consume nutrients in much higher quantities than they can reasonably obtain from foods. The best example of this is the use of vitamin E for heart disease, arthritis, and Alzheimer's treatment and prevention. The RDA for vitamin E is only about 10 IU (international units). The daily dose used in disease treatment/prevention studies is usually between 100 to 800 IU. Attempting to consume 800 IU of vitamin E from food would require the consumption of thousands of calories, leading to obesity.

Why Should I Be Careful with Supplements?

The medical community takes a rather funny approach to supplement use. The majority of physicians take dietary supplements themselves, but recommend supplements to fewer than half of their patients. It could be considered malpractice to *not* prescribe supplements to patients for certain conditions, including heart disease, anemia, osteoporosis, toxemia of pregnancy, and arthritis, as well as to prevent birth defects. And yet, physicians and physician groups regularly denounce dietary supplements as dubious or even quackery.

What's going on here? Why are doctors being so cautious, and why should you be careful as well? Aren't these little over-the-counter pills, even when ineffective, at worst harmless? Not always. We will now look at three areas of the dispute over supplements: variable quality, unsubstantiated claims, and lack of standardization in nutrient level testing.

Variable Quality of Dietary Supplements

You can walk into almost any drugstore, select a bottle of St. John's wort that claims it contains the "purest products available," spend seventeen dollars, and get something less potent than a sugar tablet. Many supplements on the shelves are completely devoid of any active ingredient. And the companies that put them on the shelves are acting completely within the law.

The FDA won't remove subpotent products from the market unless they are harmful. No independent organization, until recently (see sidebar), has routinely tested supplements for potency. If it weren't for a handful of conscientious companies that go out of their way to ensure potency and purity, dietary supplements as a whole would have been completely discredited long ago.

There are a variety of things that can go wrong when manufacturing supplements. Good manufacturing practices (GMPs) are guidelines from the FDA to help supplement companies eliminate production problems and provide safe and properly labeled products. But not all companies follow GMPs, while others try but fail. Many supplement companies receive grades from independent quality assurance reviewers on how well they perform in meeting the GMPs.

SUPPLEMENT POTENCY PEACE OF MIND, FINALLY!

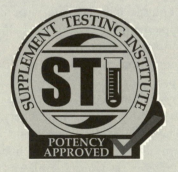

The Supplement Testing Institute (STI) is an independent organization whose mission is to allow consumers to easily identify dietary supplements that have passed postmanufacture quality assurance tests for product potency and disintegration. Think of the STI as the UL (Underwriters Laboratory) of the vitamin industry. Completely voluntary and industry-supported, supplement manufacturers choose to allow their products to be tested, and the results publicized. Consumers need only to choose products that have the following logo to know that the product they're buying meets label claims.

STI's website is at _www.supplementtesting.org_. This site also serves as a database of internal quality assurance programs for many of the industry's major companies and their grades on meeting good manufacturing practices (GMPs). Look here before buying your supplements.

Unfortunately, even with GMPs in place, things can go wrong. The only way to be completely sure you're getting the best product available is to choose companies that test *each* lot (or batch) of their supplements for potency, microbial contamination, and dissolvability.

Don't be fooled by advertising. Make sure the manufacturer proves its product is good by revealing the results of postmanufacture quality assurance testing for each lot. A listing of companies that provide these results is available at *www.supplementtesting.org*.

Unsubstantiated Claims

The second major reason why doctors have had reservations about dietary supplements is the vast barrage of unsubstantiated claims that seems to pervade the industry.

Funding for large clinical trials on supplements, the only thing that will prove they are helpful, has been much more difficult to obtain than funding for trials of pharmaceutical drugs. Lured by huge profit incentives, pharmaceutical companies can pour millions into testing their patented products, knowing that they'll recoup their costs if the drugs perform well. But you can't patent zinc, iron, or vitamin C, so supplement manufacturers are less likely to fund large studies. The National Institutes of Health get involved only if a supplement shows great promise, and have recently paid for large-scale clinical trials on glucosamine/chondroitin and St. John's wort.

Do You Really Need That Supplement?

The third significant concern many doctors have about recommending dietary supplements is that people usually take them blindly, without knowing if they really need them. Sometimes, people have too much of the nutrient in their bodies already.

Supplement overload can readily occur with vitamin B_6, iron, and the fat-soluble vitamins A, D, E, and K. Overload can also occur easily with trace minerals such as copper, selenium, manganese, and vanadium. Trace minerals, by definition, are needed in very small quantities (usually millionths of a gram). If a doctor doesn't know your deficiency or overload status of these minerals, he's less likely to recommend that you take them, for fear he may cause you harm.

There's nothing unreasonable about that. Since we monitor how other drugs affect patients, shouldn't we only recommend supplements based on levels in the body? This is common sense and good medical practice. Vitamin and mineral level testing is not a completely new or novel idea, but its scope remains limited. Here are some of the standards for nutrient screening today:

- Physicians are required to test for sodium, potassium, chloride, calcium, and phosphorus in every routine "chemistry panel," a sort of general screening for a variety of diseases.

- Since low levels of vitamins B_6, B_{12}, and folate have been associated with elevated homocysteine, doctors have been increasingly testing for these vitamins when high homocysteine levels are detected. Homocysteine is an amino acid that can cause artery disease if elevated in the blood.

- Physicians routinely check iron levels when anemia is found.

- Magnesium levels are checked in women suffering from toxemia of pregnancy and cardiac patients.

- Vitamin D levels should be checked in those with osteoporosis and osteoarthritis, especially since low levels of vitamin D contribute to accelerated progression of these two common diseases.

We believe that real progress in nutritional medicine will come when physicians have easy access to reliable nutrient testing for *all* known nutrients important for human health. Dr. Theodosakis is working to create a standard panel of fifteen to twenty nutrients that can become as widely accepted as the "chemistry panel," and check on a much broader range of nutrients. He is nearing completion on similar work for food allergy testing (see www.drtheo.com for the results).

What's the holdup? What has kept physicians from pushing for nutrient testing in the past? There are three reasons. First, most physicians are not very knowledgeable about the potential benefits of such testing.

Second, the costs at the current time seem prohibitive, especially for the patient, who must pay for nutrient testing outside of the "normal" five or six tests. A single vitamin B_6 test, for example, can cost over $100 at some labs.

The third obstacle is that there is not any agreed-upon, standard method of testing. Tests from some labs, using methods like hair analysis, have been shown to be quite unreliable. Once valid and reliable methods are agreed upon, the next step is to offer these tests in large volume to reduce the costs. The "chemistry panel" tests routinely performed by doctors have dropped in cost from over $100 to about $5 with widespread use. It is conceivable that testing for all twenty-five known essential nutrients could cost in the $25 to $50 range someday, maybe cheap enough for the HMOs to embrace.

What Supplements Should I Take?

Now that we've discussed why doctors have been traditionally wary of recommending supplements, one issue remains: What should you take? Like a good diet, the prescription for an optimal supplement regimen must be very specific. No single recommendation works for everyone. However, there are some key guidelines to follow, *provided you do not have any major medical problems*. Appendix C will give you additional information on supplementing if you have a major medical condition.

- Don't take supplements without consulting your doctor. Just because they are available over the counter doesn't mean they are 100 percent safe for everyone.

- Do not take any supplements containing iron (this would include most multivitamins) without a blood test to check your iron level. The best screening test for iron is usually a test known as "ferritin level."

- Pick supplements that resemble what you would find in food. The most effective supplements are those that provide the full spectrum of nutrients in a particular group. For example, beta-carotene, one of about forty carotenoids important for health, has proven to create problems when taken by itself, possibly because it interferes with absorption of other important carotenoids. Mixed carotenoids, which often contain alpha- and beta-carotene, lutein, lycopene, ß-crypto-xanthine, zeaxanthine, and others, are the preferred form for supplemental use. Likewise, vitamin E should be taken in a "mixed form" since the dl-alpha form of vitamin E alone pales in benefit to the complete vitamin E group. In nature, foods contain the mixture, not the individual component alone, and foods outperform supplements in most cases.

- Determine your calcium intake. In general, most adult men and women need about 1,200 and 1,500 mg of calcium per day, respectively. Most of us get 300 mg of calcium from non-dairy foods every day, and each serving of skim or 1-percent milk, low-fat yogurt, reduced-fat cheese, calcium-fortified orange juice, or tofu made with calcium has about 300 mg of calcium. So it's really a simple matter to calculate your calcium needs.

  Multiply your average number of servings of dairy products per day by 300. Add 300 to the sum. Then subtract that total from the number 1,200 if you are a man, and 1,500 if you are a woman. If the difference is greater than zero, take that many milligrams of calcium. Use calcium carbonate if you are under sixty-five, and calcium citrate if you are over sixty-five. Users of acid blockers like Zantac, Pepcid, Tagamat, Prolisec, or Prevacid should also use calcium citrate. Please note that calcium carbonate requires stomach acid to be properly absorbed.

- If you are taking calcium supplements, consider taking magnesium as well. To figure the proper dosage in milligrams, divide your calcium dose by three.

- Choose a multivitamin. The ideal multivitamin contains the following: vitamin A: no more than 5,000 IU, preferably in the form of mixed carotenoids (alpha- and beta-carotene, lutein, lycopene, ß-cryptoxanthine, zeaxanthine, others); B-complex: B_1 1.5–3.0 mg, B_2 1.7–3.4 mg, B_3 20–40 mg, B_6 2–4 mg, folate 400 mcg, B_{12} 100–250 mcg; C (includes citrus bioflavonoids) 60–180 mg; D 400–600 IU; E (mixed tocopherols) 100–400 IU.

  Remember to determine your iron status first. If your iron (ferritin) level is normal or high, do not take any supplements containing iron.

- Consider a low-dose multimineral product. Look for a product that includes the following trace minerals: boron, chromium, copper, manganese, molybdenum, selenium, vanadium, and zinc. Calcium and magnesium are not considered to be trace minerals because you require much larger quantities (see above).

- Consider additional antioxidants. Choices include more vitamin C (a mixed form like citrus bioflavonoids), mixed vitamin E (100–400 IU mixed tocopherols), selenium (100–200 mcg), pycnogenol (25–100 mg), grape seed extract, CoQ-10 (30–50 mg), alpha lipoic acid (50–100 mg), glutathione (250–500 mg), green tea extract, and N-acetylcysteine (600–1,200 mg). Keep antioxidant supplements in a cool, dark place.

- Consider additional essential oils. Omega-3 fatty acids are a form of "good" fat that is often missing from the Americans' diets. Consider crushed flax seeds (1–2 teaspoons per day) or flax oil capsules (1,000–4,000 mg per day). Flax oil is a great source of omega-3 because it's free of heavy metals, which are present in some fish. Keep flax and flax supplements in the refrigerator or freezer to prevent spoilage.

- Remember that these supplement recommendations are for people without any major medical problems. Adjustments to the regimen should be performed with the aid of a nutrition-savvy physician or registered dietitian. Changes to these recommendations, if any, and updates on nutrient level testing will be posted at Dr. Theodosakis's website, *www.drtheo.com*.

How Does Exercise Aid Prevention?

Did you know that you have the perfect body? Even if you aren't satisfied with its appearance, your body is still *perfectly* adapted to meet the physical demands you place on it. If you are a jogger, your body has become fit enough to meet the demands of your jogging.

If you haven't been exercising, but have been busy taking care of your work, home, and children, you probably have a fitness level to match. That's why you become easily winded with even moderate aerobic activity. Worst of all, if you're bedridden for three weeks, your fitness level drops to meet the very low demands of lying in bed. Indeed, your fitness may drop so low from inactivity that you can find it very difficult just to be able to walk a few steps to the bathroom.

This happens because our bodies evolved at a time when food wasn't so easy to get. Instead of burning energy to keep all our muscles primed, our bodies "learned" to only expend energy on those muscles and systems that were in constant demand. That was good for our ancestors, but isn't so good for us. Today, we have to use it or lose it.

You may have a decent energy level, but you will never maintain your fitness in the long run without "pushing" yourself a few days per week with exercise. Failure to get regular exercise is perhaps the most unnatural thing you can do to your health, next to smoking. Frailty and weakness in old age has less to do with the ravages of time than with your regular exercise habits, so pay attention!

The Four Components of Preventive Exercise

We've all heard of the importance of aerobic exercise, and many of us have heard how strength training does much more than create impressive-looking muscles. But no complete exercise program should stop there. Flexibility training will help prevent some of the most common problems associated with aging. The fourth component of an exercise program, agility and balance training, is often neglected, but terribly important. We will discuss the benefits of these four components one at a time.

All of the volumes that have been written on the importance of continuous aerobic exercise can be boiled down to one piece of advice: Do something aerobic for at least thirty minutes three times a week. It's hard to overstate the benefits of aerobic exercise. It burns calories and fat, lowers your blood pressure, reduces stress, and boosts your immune system, among many other things.

What is aerobic exercise? Any type of continuous activity that uses large muscle groups, causes your heart rate to increase, and causes your breathing to quicken can be considered aerobic exercise. Depending on your starting fitness level, brisk walking, swimming, biking, dancing, hiking, racket sports, and more than a dozen other exercises fit this category. If you're new to aerobic exercise, or if you've been sedentary for more than a few months, be sure to get "clearance" from your doctor. This may involve a physical or even a cardiac stress test.

Strength training goes straight to the three biggest causes of frailty in old age: osteoporosis, osteoarthritis, and loss of muscle. When you bear weight, you stimulate your bone cells to manufacture and deposit more minerals, thereby strengthening the bone. That makes strength training both a prevention and treatment for osteoporosis, a softening of the bones (more osteoporosis interventions can be found in appendix C).

Strength training also helps those suffering from osteoarthritis, a disease of the joints, by keeping the muscles surrounding the joints toned. Loss of muscle tone causes more force to be directed toward the joint cartilage, rather than being dissipated through the muscles. Even a low-impact activity like walking involves enough force to tear the major ligaments in the knee. Only the opposing force of our thigh muscles prevents this from happening. Strong, toned muscles can save our joint cartilage from the strain and pressure that, over time, causes osteoarthritis.

Finally, strength training allows you to keep your muscle as you age. After we hit thirty-five, we lose, on average, six to seven pounds of muscle per decade. This decrease in muscle mass causes us to become weaker and results in a lowered metabolic rate, which in turn can lead to weight gain. You need your muscle to be able to burn calories, a fact that too many "crash diets" ignore.

While strength training tones our muscles and bones to be able to handle weight, flexibility exercises help our bodies hold it all together. If we remain flexible, our ability to distribute the force of weight and impact over a wide area, or "biomechanics," can remain intact well into old age. Lose that flexibility, and chronic pain can show up in unexpected places. For example, people with tight hamstring and hip flexor muscles are likely to develop long-term lower back pain, often caused by osteoarthritis in the lower spine.

The most common and simple way to stay flexible is to stretch. Warm up with some light aerobic activity, move slowly into a stretch, and hold it for ten seconds or more. If you find a particular stretch difficult, it probably means that muscle group needs your particular attention. Stretching should be done for at least five to ten minutes three to five times per week.

Finally, no exercise program is complete without attention to agility (your stability while moving) and balance (your stability while standing still). Like all other abilities, we lose agility and balance if we don't practice them often. But unlike loss of muscle tone, for example, agility and balance can slip away slowly and subtly. Before we know it, we have lost the ability to perform even simple feats of balance, such as putting on our socks and shoes while standing on one foot.

If we lose that ability, we are more likely to experience dangerous falls when we are older. In fact, the number-one cause of injury deaths for those over seventy-five is falls. For those under seventy-five, most injury deaths are caused by motor accidents. Loss of agility becomes a vicious circle when it leads to a loss of confidence and the exclusion of ever more activities, but the solutions can be surprisingly simple.

At home, you can practice "tandem walking," placing one foot in front of the other as if you were on a tightrope. Standing on one leg and holding the pose can also help. You may feel silly, but take these simple drills seriously. More involved agility and balance exercises include dance, martial arts, yoga, and most racket sports.

Those are the four major types of exercise that, if included in your exercise plan, will result in the total fitness you need to prevent common diseases of old age. But too many of us come up against physical and psychological barriers to exercise that allow us to slip into a pattern that ignores the benefits of prevention. We'll talk next about how to stay on track.

How Do I Stick with the Program?

Our busy lives build both physical and psychological barriers to exercise. Here are some tips that may help you become as regular with your exercise as you are with brushing your teeth.

If you feel you have no time for exercise:

- Make your exercise session a top priority, an appointment that just can't be broken. It's that important. Don't say you are just too busy; if United States presidents can make time for exercise, you can as well.

- Exercise first thing in the morning, before the "urgencies" of daily life get in the way. Once your exercise is done for the day, nothing can take it away.

- If that doesn't work, use your lunch break for exercise. You can save time for your workout by packing your lunch or ordering something in advance and picking it up after you exercise. Consider extending your lunch break to accommodate your workout, making up the time by coming in early or staying late.

- Try to find a way to turn your commute into an exercise session. If you can't walk or bike to work, consider parking or getting off the bus or train a few blocks from your destination so you can do some extra walking.

- Use stairs instead of escalators and elevators. The increased activity will add up to significant health benefits over the years.

- Combine your activities. Listen to books on tape while exercising or have "walking meetings" with business colleagues. Consider taping your favorite shows to watch while exercising. This will give you something to look forward to when it's time to work out.

- Make exercise part of your social life. Team sports such as softball are great for this. Too often our social activities revolve around eating rather than exercise.

- Delegate your responsibilities. Get your spouse and children to share your chores. Don't try to do it all yourself.

- Consider a "babysitting exchange" with other parents in the neighborhood. One parent can watch the kids while the others exercise.

- Let your kids exercise with you. Biking, hiking, swimming, and exercise classes that allow older children to participate are all good choices.

Don't limit yourself to only one exercise plan. It's a guarantee for failure, because you can never predict when your daily schedule might change. For this reason it is always wise to prepare an exercise plan A and plan B. For example, plan A may include going to the gym four times each week to complete thirty minutes of aerobics and twenty minutes of weight training. If for some reason you are unable to get to the gym, you can switch to plan B, which might involve using your stair stepper and free weights at home.

If motivation is your main issue:

- Always have both outdoor and indoor options for exercise.

- Consider seasonal activities to prevent boredom and monotony.

- Use the "five minute rule." If you're having trouble getting motivated, make yourself exercise for just five minutes. If you still feel unmotivated after five minutes, quit. You probably need the rest. But most of the time five minutes is all it takes to turn your motivation on.

- Use a partner or trainer to hold you accountable. You'll have increased motivation if you pay for a trainer or your friend is waiting for you to show up.

- Choose sporting activities that take your mind off the exercise. Make it fun. Ride a bike through a beautiful park or play a competitive sport. The hours will fly by.

- Remember that vigorous daily activities like gardening, mowing the lawn, chopping wood, or walking the kids to school can be part of a physically active lifestyle.

- Finally, don't get caught up in the all-or-nothing syndrome. While maintaining a full and regular exercise routine is always best, don't forget about the need to remain psychologically connected to your commitment. Can't make it to the gym? Do a couple of sets of arm exercises before you get dressed. Knowing that you did even a little instead of letting it slide can keep you motivated.

How much exercise is enough exercise? Only you can answer this question. It's not about how much time you spend exercising, it's about the results. If you are satisfied with the results, you are doing enough. If you feel you aren't making progress, you have to either do more or increase the intensity of your exercise.

Exercise is for everyone, not just for people who want to look their best. It's a powerful weapon in the fight against the effects of aging. It's a preventive investment, and it will pay off now and for decades to come. It's the closest thing we have to the fountain of youth.

How Do Sleep and Rest Help Prevention?

Can't sleep? You're not the only one. Forty-five million Americans regularly suffer from sleep problems, and the numbers are continuing to grow. Still, most medical schools devote little attention to the subject, and even though many creative and simple treatments exist, sleeping pills are still the preferred treatment. In fact, more prescriptions are written for sleeping pills than any other medication except birth control pills.

Sleep problems can create a wide range of other health problems, including depression, lowered immunity, decline in memory and cognitive abilities, low energy level, and low appetite. Beyond that, there is evidence that chronic sleep problems can actually shave years off our lives.

Normal, healthy sleep follows a certain pattern. Each night's rest involves five or six cycles of ninety minutes each, for a total of seven and a half to nine hours. Each cycle involves four stages, progressing from light sleep at stage one to deep sleep at stage four and back again. Rapid eye movement (REM) occurs after we cycle back from stage four. By the end of the night, our sleep becomes more "shallow," with stages three and four dropping out. When doctors look at sleep problems, they use these stages to figure out exactly where the problem occurs. So far, they have found eighty-six different types of sleep disorder.

Sleep problems can be caused or exacerbated by a host of contributing factors. The most common factors affecting sleep are stress, worries, depression, misuse of sleeping pills, alcohol, tobacco, caffeine, medical problems, and aging. Age-related changes include menopause, depression, metabolic changes, multiple medications, and a decrease in the natural production of melatonin (a brain hormone produced by the pineal gland).

Sleep problems may also be symptomatic of one of many other medical problems or diseases, which is why your sleep habits are an important part of your medical history. Use the Sleep Report form in appendix A before your doctor's appointment if you have any sleep problems, no matter how small. The form should be filled out every morning for at least seven days in order to give the doctor a reasonably informative history.

Once your sleep problem has been properly diagnosed it's important to participate in good *sleep hygiene*. These are behaviors that make sure your sleep is deep, quality rest that leaves you feeling great when you wake up. Here are some simple but important steps to get you sleeping better in just a few short days:

- Make sure your bedroom is conducive to sleep. Check your mattress, sheets, pillows, and overall bedroom environment for not only physical comfort, but emotional comfort as well. For example, surround yourself with pictures of loved ones, pleasant artwork, or plants that emit a soothing aroma.

- Keep the climate in your bedroom comfortable, but slightly cooler than normal. The combination of darkness and cool temperatures actually stimulates the brain's production of a series of hormones that will initiate the desire for sleep.

- Make sure you do not have a television in your bedroom. TV is one of the great sleep destroyers of the twentieth century.

- Don't bring work into your bedroom. Work will just cause your mind to race when it should be winding down.

- If you wake up in the middle of the night, don't fight it. Give yourself ten to fifteen minutes to fall asleep; but if you don't, leave your bedroom. Don't come back until you feel sleepy again. Don't worry about becoming more awake. If you haven't been able to sleep, there's no use lying in bed. In fact, lying in bed without sleeping can cause anxiety that makes it even harder to sleep. Doctors have a name for this: *conditioned insomnia.*

- Use white noise if you need to block out other sounds. Smoothly running fans or a tape playing nature sounds can block out a neighbor's radio or even a snoring partner.

- Use aromatherapy if your problem is related to tension. Aromatherapy's potential is quite promising and is currently under study at several universities for its effects on sleep. Experiment with several different candles and incenses until you find a scent that has a soothing effect.

- *Don't look at your clock until morning.* If you obsess about the time, you will only make matters worse. Cover your clock up, put it in a dresser, or something, anything. Just don't think about the time when you are fighting insomnia.

- Maintain a regular pattern. Your body needs this pattern to produce hormones and cells and maintain its proper temperature. Your "circadian rhythms" can be interrupted if you stay up late one night and go to bed early the next night.

- Lower the light level in your home before you sleep. Using the dimmers on your lights or eating dinner by candlelight can create an atmosphere that will help transition your body's natural rhythms from a state of alert to a state of rest.

- Follow your exercise program. Exercise during the day helps improve the length and quality of sleep stages three and four, the deepest and most important for your immune system and general sense of restfulness.

- Avoid caffeine and tobacco. One cup of coffee can stay in your system for twenty hours after you drink it. Even if you are okay one day, changes in your body's rhythms can make caffeine or nicotine more problematic the next day. The best policy is to avoid them altogether.

- Use supplements and herbal sleep aids. Vitamins B_3 and B_{12} and the minerals calcium and magnesium have been shown to help some sleep problems. There are also a few herbal remedies you can try, like passionflower, kava kava, hops, and valerian root. Be careful with melatonin, often sold as a jet lag remedy. Most users report feeling worse after taking this synthetic version of your own sleep hormone. Always discuss what you are taking with your doctor just as you would let her know what medications you're taking.

- Establish a nighttime relaxation routine. Try taking a warm bath surrounded by scented candles. Experiment with massage, calm music, new slippers, and warm milk.

Sleep is just as important a part of your prevention program as diet and exercise. Losing even one night's sleep has implications that go well beyond the groggy feeling you have the next day. Those nights can pile up, and someday will catch up with you. You need your rest, no matter how busy you are, or how well you can function on just a few hours sleep. Always be sure to give that appointment with your pillow high priority.

What Changes Should I Make in My Environment?

All the exercise and diet plans you create won't help you combat the health hazards in your environment if you're constantly exposed to harmful substances. Your water, your air, and the noise pollution around you are all areas to watch closely. In this section, we'll explore the most common sources for harmful environmental exposure and teach you how to avoid or minimize their effects.

We have to admit that this section doesn't go far enough. Each job, lifestyle, and neighborhood has its own set of risks. Coal miners suffer disproportionately from lung diseases while farmers and construction workers, exposed to excess noise, heat, cold, vibration, and sunlight, are more likely to suffer traumatic injury. Bartenders, waiters, and waitresses are often exposed to excessive noise and secondhand smoke (and the occasional bar fight). Flight attendants, pilots, and frequent fliers are exposed to noise, time zone changes, and excessive radiation, since planes fly above much of the radiation-absorbing atmosphere. It's important to assess your own risks in your job and your home. Here, however, we will just cover the most common exposures: water, air, and noise.

Water

While it's relatively rare to get infections from public drinking water, we still get some chemical contaminants, including heavy metals, organic chemicals, and even some radioactive compounds. We hear quite a bit about lead, but by-products of water chlorination may actually be the biggest concern.

A by-product of water chlorination called MX was described in a 1997 article in the *Journal of the National Cancer Institute*. MX is probably the most carcinogenic of the chlorine by-products found in water. It has not been studied in humans, but in rats it causes cancer of the thyroid, lungs, skin, breast, liver, and pancreas. Admittedly, the rats used in studies of MX were given high doses, much higher than people would ever receive, but we do not know if people are more sensitive to MX than rats. Unfortunately, MX levels are not routinely monitored in drinking water. Formation of MX can be prevented by chlorinating water *after* filtering, a practice not currently performed at most water treatment facilities.

You may think you are safe if you don't drink municipal water. But think again—you probably shower in it. When you shower, trace amounts of the chlorination by-products chloroform and TCE escape from their dissolved liquid form and become vapors that you inhale. These vapors are called *volatile organic compounds,* or VOCs. When you drink chlorinated water, you don't get the full carcinogenic effect—the by-products are broken down during digestion and detoxified in your liver. But when you breathe them in the shower, they go directly into the bloodstream. A ten-minute hot shower exposes you to the equivalent of about two gallons of water consumed orally.

So drinking bottled water only takes care of part of the problem. In addition, bottled water can contain contaminants from its plastic container, and doesn't have the benefit of fluoride, which helps fight tooth decay and improves bone density. According to the Natural Resources Defense Council, an environmental watchdog group, bottled water is "not necessarily any safer, any better regulated or any purer than the water that comes out of the tap." The council tested one thousand samples of bottled water representing 103 brands and found that at least one-third of the brands had at least one bottle with contaminants. Many bottled waters are simply tap water that has been sent though a filter or purifier. If you have a real problem with tap water, a purification system may be the best solution.

Buying a purification system is a tricky proposition. What are your needs, and how can you meet them most economically? Here are a few important tips for getting the right kind of water purification system for your home:

- Get your water tested for dissolved solids. Most water companies will do this for free. If the level of dissolved solids is above 250 parts per million (ppm), one of the more expensive and sophisticated systems (often a multistage filter system including a carbon filter and reverse osmosis unit or a distiller) will be required to assure you get pure drinking water. Carbon and particulate filters alone will not do the job.

- Test for lead. Testing for lead is relatively cheap, and there are even some home testing kits, available in your hardware store, that are easy to use and cost about fifteen to thirty dollars. Using a do-it-yourself kit usually requires two samples of your water: a first-draw (the water that falls from the spigot immediately after it has been opened) and a purged-line (drawn after the water has run for a specified period of time). Lead values below fifteen parts per billion (ppb) for first-draw and five ppb for purged-line are considered safe.

- If you have to purify all the water you use, there's not much to choose from besides a whole-house particulate filter and carbon tank or a carbon block filter. These can be bought or rented. However, these will not purify drinking water as well as a dedicated drinking water system, but they are a decent substitute for a cost-conscious household. Rentals run about ten to twenty-five dollars per month, depending on water usage.

- Don't assume a water softener will do the trick. Water softeners don't remove organic chemical contaminants, or other toxic metals such as arsenic. Furthermore, the high levels of sodium (or potassium) used to "soften" the water can be inherently unhealthy, especially for those with certain heart problems or high blood pressure. The sodium can also pull lead from the pipes.

- If lead is your only problem, consider a filter cartridge. But be sure to change your filter frequently; a full filter cartridge can dump lead into the water if it isn't changed.

- Don't bother with small carbon filter units, such as those attached to faucets or used in pour-through pitchers. They are virtually useless.

- All purifiers need to be maintained properly. If they are not, your water may end up even more contaminated. This is a case for renting units, since maintenance is usually included in the rental charge.

- If you plan to purchase a water purifier, be sure to look for the NSF seal of approval. NSF stands for the National Sanitation Foundation, a voluntary certification program for water-treatment devices.

Air

The average person breathes almost a million gallons of air per year. If there are even small amounts of contaminants in the air where you work and live, over the course of a year your dose will become quite large. It's crucial to take the time to think about what is in your air and how it may affect you.

Tobacco smoke is one of the worst poisons you will find in any environment. As a society, we are foolish to allow smoking in any public place where nonsmokers are exposed against their will. Tobacco smoke, along with asbestos and benzene, is a group A carcinogen. Do we let people spray benzene on each other just because they like the smell? Didn't we force schools to remove asbestos to protect our children? Why should tobacco smoke be so different? If other highly addictive substances are classified as drugs and regulated by the FDA, why isn't tobacco?

From a medical standpoint, there is virtually nothing a person can do that is more stupid than using tobacco. If it weren't for the fact that the federal and state governments are so financially dependent on tobacco taxes, there would surely be a serious push to eliminate this scourge. Nevertheless, here we are, still smoking away into the twenty-first century. Keep away from tobacco smoke.

In addition, you should watch out for these other contaminants:

- Volatile organic compounds at the gas station. Pay for full-service and let the attendant fill the tank while you sit in your closed car. If you are pregnant, we cannot recommend this expensive option strongly enough. You can also use the clip or lever that keeps the pump handle on while you sit in your car, or make sure you are upwind of gas fumes while filling up.

- Dry cleaning solvents. The best way to avoid these chemicals is to hang your freshly cleaned clothes outside for a few hours before bringing them into the house. The solvents will quickly dissipate.

- Chemicals from new carpets and furniture. For those who have known sensitivities, it is a good idea to avoid exposure to new carpet or furniture for a few days while ventilating the room.

- Radon. There's a lot of hype about radon, and it may or may not be warranted. But even if it's not as bad as some people think, the stuff is radioactive and can't be good for you. Spring for the test—about thirty dollars—and find out if you are being exposed. If your home's levels are high, sealing the cracks in your foundation and improving your ventilation usually does the trick.

Carbon monoxide is common and lethal, so we will give it special attention. Carbon monoxide (CO) is an odorless, colorless gas that's produced by incomplete combustion of fuels, poorly serviced heating units, water heaters, stoves and fireplaces, paint removers containing methylene chloride, and cigarette smoke. Runners and bikers who exercise within a few feet of heavily trafficked roads can also have elevated CO levels, close to those of pack-a-day smokers. Carbon monoxide is the leading cause of death by poisoning in the United States today, accounting for about four thousand deaths annually.

Symptoms include headaches, breathing difficulties, and nausea at lower levels of intoxication. Visual disturbances, confusion, seizures, coma, and death can occur at higher exposures. Watch for these warning signs, and get the inexpensive home test. If your home's levels are high, maintenance of household appliances, smoking cessation, and improved home ventilation can solve the problem.

Overall, the key to preventing harmful exposure to airborne contaminants is ventilation. Dilution can "cure" almost all bad-air problems. Be sure to avoid tobacco smoke and any chemicals that smell "funny," like nail polish remover, solvents, bug killers, and pesticides. In the vast majority of cases a smell that seems artificial is likely to be harmful, so limit your exposure.

Noise

There's an overabundance of noise in our environment. We seem to be exposed to more noise than ever before: rush-hour traffic, emergency vehicles, loud music, airplanes, hunting and shooting, yard and lawn equipment, the whine of office equipment and fluorescent lighting. These are just some everyday sources of noise exposure that can lead to hearing loss, an epidemic in our aging society. Beyond this obvious consequence, excessive noise can lead to other serious health problems such as depressed immune systems, sleep disorders, and high blood pressure.

The solution is simple: take earplugs with you if you *must* go into a situation where you know you'll be exposed to excessive noise. The foam ones found in drugstores work well, but custom-fitted ones are the best. Most audiologists can make a wax mold of your ear canal and, for as little as $30, supply you with perfect-fitting ear plugs, comfortable even for extended use at movies, concerts, or on airplanes. For higher-intensity noise, the headphone-type of earguard may be more effective.

Save your hearing! After following the preventive guidelines in this chapter, you may need to use your ears for many decades to come!

How Does Being Connected to the Community Help?

People need people. No one can deny this, but it's a fact that too often is left out of discussions of preventive medicine. Recently, however, medical research has acknowledged that being cared for and caring for others dramatically impacts the body's rate of recovery from illness as well as the body's ability to fight disease. The healing powers of kindness, love, and intimacy are finally being considered as frontline therapies for many physical and emotional illnesses.

The life and death importance of social connectedness has been revealed in studies showing that widowers are 40 percent more likely to die in the six months after their spouse's death than other men their age. Interestingly, the widower's mortality returns to that of other men his age if he remarries or if he survives five years. A well-known study undertaken in Alameda County, California, over nine years showed that men and women who were isolated from their community, family, and friends were more than twice as likely to die as those who reported meaningful and strong relationships. Feelings of hopelessness, loss, and loneliness have repeatedly been linked with susceptibility to infectious diseases, heart disease, diabetes, arthritis, cancer, ulcerative colitis, cervical cancer, and leukemia. The case for being socially connected is strong.

Disengagement from social ties and meaningful relationships can cause feelings of passivity and apathy. Conversely, individuals who feel they have control over the circumstances of their lives show a significant increase in physical activity, intellectual pursuits, healthier eating and sleeping, and overall quality of life. The majority of people who engage in these activities grow into older age with little to no decline in memory, intellect, physical activity, sexual intimacy, and sleep. Think about it: during those times in your life when you felt good about yourself and others, didn't you find yourself more motivated to maintain healthy lifestyle habits?

We need one-on-one intimacy and we need community ties with people who share common interests and goals. How does someone begin to take the steps out of isolation and into socialization? First, it begins with you and what you care about. Ask yourself what interests you and what is important to you. For example, you might come to the conclusion that you are interested in gardening and you care about politics. Your next move would be to contact gardening clubs and political organizations. Taking the first step by reaching out is the hardest, but the most important part. People who have experienced loneliness for any length of time can find it difficult to reach out, feeling unworthy and overly self-conscious. However, pushing yourself and getting through the initial awkwardness will enable you to meet others who share your interests and your passions. Here are some suggestions of places to contact that will help bring you the meaningful friendships and activities you've been hoping for:

- Spiritual organizations

- Sports organizations like the YMCA, parks or recreation departments, and local health clubs.

- Arts and crafts organizations at museums, universities, and community colleges

- Newcomers' clubs and welcome wagons

- Hospitals, nursing homes, elementary schools, and animal shelters that offer opportunities to do volunteer work

While participation in organizations isn't a substitute for intimacy, it is a start. Making contact in and of itself creates hope and self-esteem. Positive feelings almost always lead to positive behaviors that will eventually lead you to people and places that can offer meaningful support.

By now you've probably figured out that living a long and fulfilling life means that you have to take into account your entire daily existence. Everything you eat, every activity you do, the environment in which you live, and the people you see all affect your physical and mental well-being. As you embark on your preventive program, you will begin to see that the two are completely inseparable. Once you understand this simple and irrefutable truth, you will be able to get the most out of eating right, exercising, and staying involved in the community. Prevention does more than just bring you closer to a goal that lies somewhere down the road. It pays off now, and it pays off big.

That should be enough to convince you that you should engage in prevention even if your HMO doesn't help. It's unlikely that your health insurance will offer the holistic approach that will ensure a long and healthy life. Don't expect your managed care company to manage everything. It's your life, and in the end, only you can save it.

How Can My HMO Help?

The best preventions are the ones you can do completely on your own, but you can also coax your HMO into becoming a part of your prevention team. Appendix C lists several preventive screening recommendations for common diseases. Most of these guidelines are widely recognized as standard, and no HMO should deny them. But don't let a denial from an HMO prevent you from getting the test. You may have to pay out of pocket, but it will be some of the smartest money you've ever spent.

At the beginning of this chapter, we discussed why managed care can't and won't see the benefit in offering a full array of preventive services, no matter how much sense prevention makes in the long term. But the good news is that the industry is under intense pressure to make prevention a focus. The National Committee on Quality Assurance (NCQA) takes prevention seriously, and accredits only HMOs that meet basic guidelines for screening tests like mammograms, cervical cancer screening, and eye exams for diabetics.

If your HMO has full accreditation from the NCQA, you may have noticed that your doctors really push you to get certain screenings. This is because the HMO is being graded on how much of their population gets screened. That doesn't mean you should rest easy. Even if your HMO is making a serious effort to live up to the NCQA's recommendations, they still have to balance profit against care. They may still try to get away with just the minimum, even though you deserve the best.

Starting with the top causes of death and prevalence and incidence of disease at a particular age group (you can find these in appendix B), add in your own personal medical history, your family history, and most importantly, your recent and current lifestyle habits. All of this data can be used by your doctor to estimate your personal risk profile.

Many patients are amazed to find that they have been focusing their health efforts in areas less likely to provide efficient risk reduction. Patients should not be expected to calculate or estimate their own risks; this is a job for their physician.

Make an appointment with your primary care physician with the sole goal being prevention. When you go to the appointment, don't talk about other medical problems and then get to prevention at the very end, when the doctor is out of time. Walk in and say, "Doctor, I'm here to get your help in estimating my top five risks for disease or death. I'd like to figure out if I need to make any changes in my lifestyle and if there are any screening tests or other interventions we may consider. If we have to take more than one appointment to do this, I'd be glad to come back."

Come armed with a good description of your family history, in writing. Include all of your first-degree relatives (children, parents, and siblings) and as many second-degree relatives (aunts, uncles, cousins, nieces, nephews, and grandparents) as you can get information on. List their current ages and health status. For any deaths, list the relative's age at death, the cause of death, and any major medical problems they might have had over the course of their lives. Also come armed with all your current medications in a plastic bag, a description of your current medical problems (to remind your doctor), and an honest description of your major lifestyle habits such as tobacco, alcohol, and drug use; sexual habits and risks of sexually transmitted diseases; and exercise and diet patterns. Ask the doctor if there are screening tests, or other screening interventions.

Then, after you have established the *best* strategy, find out what your HMO will cover. It's important to keep these two issues separate when talking to your doctor. Managed care's money issues may have affected his medical thinking. He may have been persuaded, directly or indirectly, to not advise patients to pursue tests they have every right to get.

You can get complete and honest answers if you let your doctor know that you will settle for no less than the best, and that you are willing to pay out of pocket if the HMO won't cover a screening that you need. This takes the pressure off the doctor to recommend only the minimum screening. Once you have a list of the best preventive treatments, you can begin to select what the HMO will pay for without any hassles, what they might pay for if you pressure them, and what they will definitely not pay for.

Your own research may uncover other tests and measures that your doctor missed, and calls to your health plan can establish whether they are covered or not. Once you have a list of your tests and measures, including things that you can do on your own and things that you can pay for out of pocket, it's time to make a schedule.

Integrate the clinical side of your preventive plan with your exercise and diet schedule. Think about all the preventive steps you are taking as part of a single process. Showing up for your screenings is just like sticking to your exercise program—it takes awareness, clear goals, and commitment to make it work.

The rewards are amazing. When a screening turns up negative, you know that it's not just due to good luck or good genes. It's a result *you* achieved by sticking to your healthy habits. If there is a positive result, you can take comfort in the fact that your doctors caught it early because you stuck to your screening schedule.

The greatest reward, however, is the years you are adding to your life. Your planning and persistence are an investment in the future. When you blow out a small forest of candles on your birthday cake, watch your grandchildren grow, and wake up feeling great at eighty-five years old, you can look back at the wise choices you made years ago with pride.

What Have I Accomplished?

Prevention can put you on a high road to health. The HMO is mostly out of the picture when you work on your prevention plans or take advantage of a nonmainstream treatment, but don't let that stop you. Managed care is good for some things, and not so good for others. It plays a crucial role when we get sick or when we are due for a clinical screening test. The rest of the time, we are on our own.

Being on our own isn't so terrible. In the world of preventive medicine, we have more choice, more possibilities, and sometimes even better results. We can be true consumers of health care, selecting what works best for us as individuals. In the world of managed care, where it is so often assumed that the same plan should work for everyone, you must be the champion of your own health.

~ 6 ~

Sick Days

Getting Well with Your HMO

QUESTIONS THIS CHAPTER ANSWERS

◆ *The test was positive. What do I do now?*

◆ *Where can I get information on medical tests?*

◆ *How do I research my condition?*

◆ *What will I find on the Internet?*

◆ *Should I seek help outside the HMO?*

◆ *How do I present my research to my doctor?*

◆ *How do I build a medical team?*

Even if you are happy with your managed care plan, you've probably had this terrifying thought: You are stuck with your HMO, which has handled most of your minor problems well enough. You've maintained a good relationship with your doctor, and you've followed a preventive treatment program. Then, after a routine screening test, your doctor delivers bad news. The test was positive: you might have an illness that threatens your life. It's at times like these that we wish we weren't in an HMO.

If you've been reading the managed care horror stories in the press, you've probably noticed a few common themes. The victim might have survived if the appeal had gone through in time. The victim might still be with us if the HMO had been better organized in getting a visit to a specialist approved. Catastrophe might have been averted if only the doctor had recognized that the presence of one disease means that he should check for another. If only the patient had been held for observation, rather than quickly discharged from the hospital. It seems like HMOs are always ready to give us another lesson in the clarity of hindsight.

What the HMO horror stories should be teaching us, however, is the value of being prepared. We used to be able to count on our hospitals to take the lead in coordinating our treatment. Every specialist and procedure you might need, and probably many you didn't need, was at your service, no questions asked. Then the HMOs started asking questions. Questioning takes time, and that means delays. Appeals take more time, and all too often there's no patient to treat by the time management is ready to care.

Take the lead from the beginning. Arm yourself with information, be ready to anticipate your HMO's questions and denials, and don't approve any procedure or treatment you don't understand.

Don't assume that your doctor knows all and knows best. There are some 25,000 medical journals in print. Around fifty of those are considered essential. No one has the time to read all this material. The hard-working indexers at MedLine, the National Medical Library's journal database, have so far collected nine million medical journal article abstracts. There's just too much to read, especially when you are a general practitioner and need to know a little bit about everything.

It's your condition and you are living with it. You can do yourself and your doctor a huge favor by just getting your feet wet in the oceans of medical information out there. In the process, you might find a new treatment, an unusual approach, or something your doctor might have missed. Many of today's doctors admit that patients often motivate them to learn about new medical advances, something that rarely happened just ten years ago.

Don't assume that your primary care physician will be the manager of your treatment program. He's got too many patients to see, and he's just one part of the managed care puzzle. He might not even know what resources are available to you through your plan. HMOs are vast, offering everything from surgery to physical therapy. Your doctor may not know where you and your condition fit in. But you can't let details slip by. Researching your condition will give you the right questions to ask your HMO, and allow you to actively manage and coordinate your own treatment.

You may be asking: "I have to do this all myself? What am I paying them for, anyway?" Well, for one thing, we are paying much less than we would if we were all on indemnity plans. By being in an HMO, some of the work that you aren't paying for now has to be done by you.

The same thing happened to gas stations. They all used to be full-service, but now if you want the cheap gas, you'll have to get out and do a little pumping yourself (just stay away from the fumes!). This is not all bad, and may even be considered a great opportunity. Shouldn't you know as much about your treatment as possible? Shouldn't you be sure that you're getting the best? Don't you want to be able to talk to your doctor about what's happening to you? Performing some basic research will give you that chance.

We've spent the first half of this book concentrating on how to talk to your doctor and how to keep from getting sick in the first place. The tips you have already received should get you through most situations, but when you have a real problem, you will have to be ready to research and manage your solutions. The chapter you are about to read will guide you through sick days with your health plan, from the point where you learn about a positive test result to the stage where you bring all the HMO's resources to focus on you. Managed care *can* make you well, but it won't do it without your help.

The Test Was Positive: What Can I Do?

Your doctor comes in with bad news. The mammogram found a lump. The blood test found high sugar levels. The typical reaction is to feel helpless or even start to panic. There's a chance you have a real problem and can do nothing about it. You feel you might have to just throw yourself on the questionable mercy of your health plan. All the power you gained learning HEAD and following a preventive medicine program is in danger of slipping away. You can't let that happen.

The first thing you have to do is stay calm. A positive test result doesn't mean it's over. It means that a plan has to be developed, or the plan you are following has to be changed. When you hear about a positive test result, the only thing to do is start preparing for the next step. Remember that you have to remain an active participant in every stage of your treatment, in every decision about your treatment. If you panic at the first sign of trouble, there's a chance the decision will be made without you. Take a deep breath, and start asking questions.

- What does this test result mean? Say you test positive for high cholesterol. We've all heard about cholesterol, but do you know exactly what it is? Do you know what processes in your body are affected by high cholesterol? Do you know why it's important to keep cholesterol levels low? Don't rely on a vague, preconceived notion about high cholesterol. Don't assume that you know all about it from the articles you've read in the newspaper. Ask questions as if you had never heard about cholesterol before.

- How does the test work? Some tests don't actually look for the cause of the disease, but your reaction to it. Most HIV screening tests, for example, can't tell if the virus is in you, but only if you are producing antibodies as a reaction to the virus. Preliminary cancer screening tests often look for features *associated with* cancer, but don't tell you if you actually have cancer. Get this information. It will help you understand where you are in the process of coming to a diagnosis, and can even help you understand how the disease works.

- How accurate is the test? No test is 100 percent accurate. The possibility of a "false positive" is always there. This explains why you may be tested twice in many cases. Of course, cost-cutting practices may incline your doctor to avoid going back for a second test. You could wind up being treated for something you don't have. Always find out what accuracy you should expect from your test.

- What could affect the test results? What are the other possible causes of a test result? Many test results can be altered by your diet, your activities, or prescription, over-the-counter, and illegal drugs— factors not related to the disease for which you were tested. One common example is poppy seeds, which can cause a positive test for narcotics; another is meat consumption or aspirin use, which can produce a positive stool test for colon cancer.

By asking these questions, you are taking an active role in *interpreting* the test results, the same thing your doctor is trying to do. Remember that doctors very, very rarely do the tests themselves. Ultrasounds are performed by trained clinicians, blood samples are sent off to laboratories. The actual work is generally beyond your doctor's control. There are several steps along the way, and many players involved. Each step and each set of hands make possible a false or misleading result, so stay alert, ask questions, and always be sure the explanations make sense to you.

We've seen tests go badly dozens of times. It's one of the most frustrating parts of this job, because even though it's out of our hands, we're the ones who have to relay the information to the patient. We can see the concern in our patients' faces, no matter how often we say that's it's not yet time to be concerned. And since we're not the ones actually performing the test, we tend to wonder ourselves how well it was done. It's a situation we have little control over. This is a time when you, the patient, can help the doctor feel more in control by asking the right questions. They are questions your doctor should be asking herself.

Dr. Feinberg remembers a tricky consultation with the parents of an infant born with "ambiguous genitalia." It's not uncommon for some children to be born with genitalia that can't be distinguished. Put simply, the doctors didn't know if the baby was a boy or a girl. To answer the first question these parents had about their child an ultrasound needed to be performed. If the ultrasound revealed ovaries, they had a girl. If not, the baby was a boy.

It should have been that simple, but the clinician taking the ultrasound misread the instructions and took an ultrasound of the abdomen rather than the pelvis. So the test results were meaningless. Making matters worse, the clinician had produced an ultrasound that gave a glimpse of the baby's heart, where he observed potential abnormalities in the baby's ventricles. Now Dr. Feinberg had to explain to the parents not only that the sex of their child was still unknown, but that they had to go back again to check out this possible abnormality in the heart.

Forty-eight hours later, the tests were done correctly—and everything was fine. The heart was in good shape, and the pelvic ultrasound showed that the baby was a girl. But it had taken two unnecessary days before the parents could settle down. Dr. Feinberg was frustrated, a bit angry, and felt like he had little control over the situation; fortunately, the parents made all the difference. They didn't panic, they didn't blame him for the mistake, and they asked the right questions. By being active and present during the consultations, they helped Dr. Feinberg focus on the problem and get his job done.

Patients can also help by asking themselves what might cause certain test results. Dr. Theodosakis remembers one patient who tested positive for blood in his stool. There weren't any other symptoms, and nothing in the basic exam that suggested a problem. When mysteries like this come up, often the only answer seems to be the initiation of more invasive procedures—internal examinations that are unpleasant for the doctor and the patient alike. A passive patient would have silently undergone these procedures, but this patient thought to offer his own hypothesis. A hunter, as he reminded Dr. Theodosakis, his favorite dish was duck's blood soup. This culinary peculiarity sounded like a good explanation for the test result, so Dr. Theodosakis asked his patient to stay off the soup for a time. When they ran the test again a couple of weeks later, it came back negative, proving them right.

Strange tales aside, you should take your test result seriously. It's always telling you something; the trick is to determine what. To do this means that, above all, you have to keep a clear mind. Don't panic—there's work to be done. Doing that work will not only protect you against HMO cost-cutting practices, it will help you stay calm and objective. Gathering information can go a long way toward easing your fears.

So when you get a positive test result, start taking notes. What are the other possible causes of the result? You need to know all your doctor can tell you about the disease he suspects. Write down the medical name of the disorder exactly as the doctor says it. Ask him if he thinks he knows what stage you are in. Find out what follow-up tests are required. Write those down as well.

You will need to talk to someone before you start your research. If your doctor doesn't have time at that moment, or thinks you should

RESOURCES ON MEDICAL TESTS

A good place to start your research is by getting information on how your doctor knows what he knows. There are several excellent resources that explain medical tests in plain English. Here are a few:

The Yale University School of Medicine Patient's Guide to Medical Tests
Houghton Mifflin, 1997

Everything You Need to Know about Medical Tests
Springhouse Publishing Company, 1997

The Encyclopedia of Medical Tests
Michael B. Brodin
Pocket Books, 1997

The Diagnostic Procedures Handbook
at http://beWELL.com/dph/index.shtml

wait until he is certain, get a second appointment. You will want to understand what anatomical system the disease affects. You will want to know what you should expect to happen next. You will also want to know who the experts are in the related medical field.

Who are the best specialists for this disorder? Which hospitals are pioneering research in this field of medicine? Make sure that your doctor understands that you still trust his judgment—you are just seeking information. It doesn't matter if the plan covers these experts or not. Do not let financial issues guide your care at this time. You don't want to limit your best options just because the doctor assumes that you are interested in the most cost-effective approach. Just let him know that you are the sort of patient who likes to understand things, and that seeking out the experts is an important piece of the puzzle.

By the time you leave the office, you should have a good idea of what your condition, or possible condition, is and what the next steps are. You are ready to start digging for more information. Basic medical research isn't hard, and can help you see your problem in a new light. If you do a thorough job, you can then use your findings to help your HMO see the same light.

How Do I Research My Condition?

By asking your doctor direct questions, you have already started your research. By listening closely, and writing down what he says, you have taken the first step toward understanding what's happening to you. It really is only the first step. We used to be able to count on long consultations—visits we could attend completely unprepared. In the typical office visit, the patient asks only four questions. That's far too few. How many questions would you ask when buying a car? How well would you prepare yourself before going to the dealer? Well, your health care is surely much more important than a new car. Thanks to managed care, only the best-informed patient with the best questions will get the best care.

We are lucky, however, that at the same time the nature of medical research is changing. You've heard of the information revolution, and you may have wondered if it really is as dramatic as our technology companies would have us believe. Well, as far as access to medical information goes, there is no question. If you have access to a phone, a computer with a modem, or a public library, you have access to more medical information than even doctors themselves did just ten years ago.

Everyone, it seems, is interested in telling you about your health. Evening newscasts make a point of beating the *New England Journal of Medicine* to press on even minor breakthroughs. Business magazines like *Forbes* and *Fortune* provide medical news even when it's not clear what it might have to do with business. And the Internet is

SOME GENERAL RESEARCH TIPS

- Go from the general to the specific. Your first searches will be based around your diagnosis. Then you will want to look at associated conditions that may arise from your diagnosis. Then proceed to your possible treatments.

- Go from the most accessible material to the more difficult material. You will get lost if you begin your research with the *New England Journal of Medicine*. Start instead with information sources created specifically for patients.

- On the other hand, don't be intimidated by medical journal articles, even if you can't understand everything in them. Each one will have an introduction and conclusion that should make sense to you. Focus on these parts. Then ask your doctor or another expert to explain the hard parts.

- As you collect material, pay attention to when it was published. As you read, go from the oldest material to the most recent. Since medical science is moving so fast, you should stick with recent material, unless you find a seminal, unrefuted source.

- Consider the source. You should question any material from companies that stand to profit from their own advice. Put most of your faith and efforts into material that comes from nonprofit associations, government agencies, and consumer groups. Ask yourself: "Why was this written? Who's the intended audience? What purpose does it serve?"

- Seek diverse sources. Even if two articles are saying pretty much the same thing, keep copies of both. They may help convince an administrator somewhere down the line.

- Keep track of references. Good research always leads to more material, so be ready to write down new sources as you learn about them.

- Keep a list of terms you don't understand. You can look these up later.

swimming with health information (and misinformation) delivered via websites, newsgroups, and electronic mailing lists.

The biggest obstacle you will face as your own medical researcher will be information overload, not an information deficit. Fortunately, this obstacle is much easier to overcome. Rather than learning how to dig, you will just have to teach yourself how to be organized. You will need to be able to separate outdated, unhelpful, or false information from what is really helpful. Foundations, associations, government agencies, and private companies have already done the hard work for you. Essentially, all you have to do is read carefully and pay attention.

How Do I Keep from Getting Overwhelmed?

Back in chapter 4, when we introduced you to HEAD, we explained that being organized during your visit is the best way to avoid the rambling statements that infuriate doctors. You learned that there was no mystery to communicating your symptoms, that the answer is simple—proper organization. The same goes for your research. If you start with a plan, you can't go wrong.

First: What Do I Need to Know?

You will have questions, so write them down. Let's take an example. A patient, Marion, calls her doctor's office to find that her glucose tolerance test has indicated a high blood sugar level. More tests are needed, but Marion's symptoms, along with this result, suggest that she has diabetes. Marion decides, wisely, not to wait for more tests to begin her research. Rather than worry, she decides to learn.

Marion takes pen to paper and writes her questions down. What is diabetes? What type of diabetes could this be? What tests will confirm or rule out this diagnosis? What are the possible treatment plans? What are the possible complications? What diseases might be associated with diabetes? What specialist or specialists should I see? Is there anyone particularly good in my area? What drugs are involved in treatment, and what are the possible side effects? Finally, she asks if her plan will cover everything she needs.

Marion takes a look at her questions and realizes that they can be divided into three groups.

- What do I have?
- What should my treatment goals be?
- Who can be a part of my treatment team?

She's already turned a large number of questions into a more manageable group of questions. In just a few minutes, she's gotten herself organized and ready to move on to the next step.

Second: Where Will I Find This Out?

Marion now thinks about how she will find answers to her questions. She starts a second list, with her doctor's name at the top. When Marion goes in to see him again, she will put some of these questions to him. She remembers those patient information pamphlets in his office, each one addressing a specific disease. There's another source she won't have to go far to get. There are bound to be books on the topic, and the local bookstore has a good health section, so she starts a list of books to read. That reminds her that she recently read an article about the wealth of health information on the Internet. Better start a page listing websites. What else? There must be foundations devoted to diabetes research. Marion decides to find them, and starts a separate page for foundations and associations.

Marion has never gone to another doctor for a second opinion, but she figures this would be the right time. She's not sure her health plan will cover this visit, but she feels it's important enough to put an outside doctor on her "sources" list. Chances are her plan won't cover the visit, but she's right—this is important. If you are ever diagnosed with a serious illness, it's always a good idea to get advice outside the health plan. Some plans will pay for a second opinion; even if your plan doesn't, you should be ready to pay for a consultation yourself. You shouldn't have to pay out of pocket for your treatment, but you should be ready to pay for information.

Third: Do I Have All I Need?

As Marion sifts through her research material, she finds some of her answers right away, but notices that as she learns more about diabetes, new questions keep popping up. For example, she learns that osteoporosis is common in people with diabetes, but also that researchers aren't sure why. Now she has a few new questions.

As you do your research, keep referring back to your list of questions. Mark off questions you feel you have answered. Put new questions in each of the three broad categories you began with. You are getting closer to finding the keys to your care, but they won't fit in the lock unless you stay organized. As Marion learns about her risks for osteoporosis, she puts one question—"What is osteoporosis?"—in her

---

HELP OUTSIDE THE HMO's WALLS:
THE INFORMATION-ONLY CONSULTATION

When you are faced with a chronic or life-threatening illness, it's only natural to wonder if your HMO is doing everything right. Paying for an information-only visit to an off-plan specialist should cost two hundred dollars or less, and will buy you valuable information, not to mention peace of mind. Here are some things to keep in mind for your visit.

- Find the best. Ask your doctor who is the best person in your area. If you don't feel comfortable asking your doctor, ask around at a teaching hospital. You can also look at books like *America's Best Hospitals* from *U.S. News and World Report*, which lists hospitals by area and illness.

- Be sure to ask for an information-only consultation. You don't want treatment, and you don't want tests. These would make the visit considerably more expensive.

- Don't go to the consultation until you have made a good start on your research. This way, you will have more direct questions to ask.

- Bring copies of your tests and medical records. Most of the time, it's only necessary to bring records from the last couple of doctor visits. Lab results, radiology, and pathology reports along with your doctor's dictated medical notes and letters are key records to include. These records will allow the consultant to quickly learn what has been done to arrive at your diagnosis and treatment plan.

- During your visit, use HEAD to introduce yourself: "I'm a thirty-one-year-old white caretaker, recently diagnosed with type I diabetes. I'm here for an information-only consultation." Be sure to give the exact diagnosis.

- Be sure to cover your HMO's plan for treating your disease during your consultation. Be ready to explain what medications and other treatments they have prescribed. Ask if they've left anything out.

"Illness" category. She adds "How can it be monitored?" to her "Treatment" category, and adds "Specialist—title unknown" to her list of team members. When she learns what the specialist who treats this disorder is called, she will fill in that blank.

Fourth: How Can I Assess This Information?

When you feel you are nearly done, take a look at what you have learned. Try to take the facts you have gathered about your illness and turn them into goals. Sure, you have learned a lot, but how does it apply to your situation? Phrasing what you know about the illness in terms of goals will bring it all back to you and help you assess your condition.

Time to go back to HEAD for a quick self-assessment. Marion reviews her own medical history in light of what she has learned about her condition. She remembers that she suffers from flu almost every year. During her research, she found out that flu can be deadly to people with diabetes. Her goal: to avoid those annoying yearly bouts with the flu at all costs. When she reviews her social history, she looks at all the sugar she's been eating. Now she knows that she will have to avoid those foods. Her goal: establish a safe and enjoyable diet.

Using HEAD after you have done your research is the best way to get it all organized in a way that will make sense to both you and your doctor. You will also bring all the facts and advice you have gathered to focus on *you*—you haven't been doing all this research just for the sake of knowledge. But above all, you will set yourself up for the final and most important step: making a decision.

Fifth: How Do I Decide on the Best Treatment?

This is the goal of all your research. Remember that treatments can include a variety of interventions including: supplements, drugs, surgery, and lifestyle changes, to name a few. You will want to know answers to questions like these: What are the risks involved in my treatment? What are the benefits? Are the treatments preventive or reactionary? Do they treat the causes or just the symptoms? Also keep in mind that you may have to leave your health plan for some treatments, particularly the ones your plan calls "alternative," "complementary," or "experimental."

Based on your research, make a shopping list of treatments. Be sure to write down the source of your information—where you learned about the treatment. As you go back for more material or talk your treatment plan over with your doctor, some potential treatments will drop off your list. Perhaps you aren't at a stage where a certain treatment is appropriate, or perhaps another treatment you learned about has recently been discredited. But cross a treatment off your list only if you are sure that you don't need it. With a list of treatments in hand, it becomes easy to build the list of medical professionals you will need to see. These professionals will become a medical team that you will put together. We'll discuss how later in this chapter.

Marion is by now defining many of the terms of her treatment. She already knew that she would have to change her diet as a part of managing her diabetes. But she didn't know that exercise could go right to the heart of the problem, lowering her glucose levels by improving her body's sensitivity to insulin. So Marion resolves to ask her doctor about an exercise program. Having learned about the risks of flu, she resolves to get flu shots every year. Eye exams are also on her list of treatments. At her next visit to her doctor, she will be ready with a number of important questions, and ready to understand the answers.

Following these five steps will help keep you focused on your problem as you wade into the medical information pool. Doing research can be incredibly exciting. You are making discoveries. You are learning things that maybe even your doctor didn't know. And you are putting yourself in a strong position, one where it will be hard for your HMO to deny you care.

I'm Ready to Start: Where Do I Go First?

Marion had the right idea by starting with more general and easy-to-understand material. She picked up a few pamphlets from the doctor's office, which gave her an overview and ideas about where to go for more information. Comprehensive medical reference books, like the *Merck Manual of Medical Information, Home Edition,* one of our favorites, are also valuable general information sources. You will want to use these as starting points. Some of your general questions will be answered right away, but don't stop here. If you stay alert, you will find yourself asking new questions.

Check the references to your general sources. See if any of the journal articles mentioned apply to you. As you read, be sure to pay attention to questions the source can't answer. For example, Marion found that osteoporosis is associated with diabetes, but research hadn't determined why. Is there more recent research on this topic? Would it be helpful? Follow leads in your reference book to the most current articles.

Keep a list of authorities. Who is pioneering research in this area? Citations in your reference book might tell you. Add foundations, associations, and networks to your list of authorities. When you are nearly done with your research, you will be able to go straight to the source with direct questions.

As we turn ever more frequently to the Internet for information, we may be tempted to forget about books. We shouldn't. Internet sources can be as good, as true, and as useful as printed sources, but rarely do they go as deep as books. Looking things up on the Web isn't always as practical or as effective as looking them up in a book. If you have a chronic illness, you will want to use both. Start building a library of useful books, then use the Internet to get the latest information.

If Marion uses Amazon.com to find a book on diabetes, she will be faced with a list of over 1,300 titles. How can she narrow this down? First, she should look for the recognized authorities. The American Diabetes Association has several books on different aspects of her illness. She should look for books that have gone through several editions. She should always stick with publications that are up-to-date. She can always ask her primary care physician or specialist which ones are best. But for the most part, she will find that the basic information in each book is "tried and true." For the very latest news and information, she will want to go online.

What Will I Find on the Internet?

What you can find on the Internet is nothing short of amazing. So far, it's the only medium that can really keep up with the pace of medical science, and even better, most of it is absolutely free. If you haven't ventured onto the Internet before, this is a good time to begin. Find someone who knows how it works. They can explain the basics and get you started in just a few minutes. If you don't have a connection at home or work, just about every public library now has at least one computer terminal devoted to the Internet. You can save time, money, and a great deal of anxiety by taking advantage of this powerful research tool.

When you go online, it's more important than ever to remember to stay focused. The World Wide Web is vast and intricately linked, and it's easy to get distracted by an entry or article that will take you away from a site that could be more useful. Within minutes, your carefully crafted research plan could be completely forgotten. Always keep this original plan in mind, and don't start randomly following links.

Let's follow Marion as she starts the online segment of her research. Marion first selects a few general health pages to check out. She picks MedHelp International (www.medhelp.org), HealthFinder (www.healthfinder.gov), and MedicineNet (www.medicinenet.com). The suffixes—org, gov, com—tell her that she's likely looking at one website run by a nonprofit, one that's from a government agency, and one that's commercial. An "edu" suffix will tell her that she's looking at a website from a school.

Each of these websites allows Marion to search for "diabetes." Since these sites are geared toward patients, she will get a manageable number of "hits"—references to her search query. At MedHelp, Marion gets a list of articles on diabetes. A few articles give overviews, and one is from the National Institutes of Health. Marion opens this one, skims it, and prints it. Further down the list there's an article from the Department of Heath and Human Services on why people with diabetes should avoid raw seafood. She prints this article as well, glad that she has uncovered this important information, but not so pleased that she will have to give up her sushi.

Further down, there's an article on diabetic retinopathy—a serious eye condition associated with her diagnosis. She learns quite a bit from this short article. There's an anatomical drawing explaining the problem, and the author points out that she might not experience symptoms until it's too late. She learns that the National Eye Institute is conducting research into this problem. This institute gets added to her list of authorities.

Marion's list of authorities gets even longer after she visits HealthFinder, a project of the Department of Health and Human Services. Here, her search for "diabetes" gives her a list of seventy-seven web resources and associations, including a few she never would have thought of on her own. For example, the Wound Care Institute, "for the advancement of wound healing and diabetic foot pathology," reminds Marion that her condition can even affect her feet. She'd better make an appointment with a podiatrist to learn about preventive foot care for diabetics.

At this point, Marion is beginning to understand that her doctor wasn't being lax in not telling her everything. There is just too much. He is, of course, a generalist, and has to know a little about everything. It's understandable that he missed the DHHS's warnings on seafood. At the same time, Marion is becoming confident that she can find out these things for herself.

After looking at the general and specific sites geared toward patients, Marion feels ready to tackle the material geared toward professionals. This is where the most recent, leading-edge information can be found. Two collections will prove particularly useful: The National Guideline Clearinghouse (www.guideline.gov) and MedLine, the journal database of the National Library of Medicine.

The National Guideline Clearinghouse is a project of the Department of Health and Human Services and the Agency for Health Care Policy and Research in partnership with the American Medical Association and the American Association of Health Plans. If you visit this site, be sure to keep in mind that it was intended for professionals, and you should seek professional help in interpreting what you find. The purpose of the project is to collect and compare various recommended guidelines for diagnosis and treatment of disease. The guidelines that you will find there come from various organizations, not necessarily the ones named above.

Marion heads to the National Guideline Clearinghouse and enters "diabetes" into the search area. She gets sixty-two hits, and selects one that seems most general: "Standards of Medical Care for Patients with Diabetes Mellitus" from the American Diabetes Association. The first thing she notices is that the recommendations are set up like HEAD, with recommendations to get specific parts of the patient's history, such as rapid weight fluctuations. Marion checks these to make sure she and her doctor didn't miss anything. Since Marion read chapter 4 and knew how to work effectively with her physician, they didn't.

As Marion scrolls through this article, she finds confirmation for much of what she's already learned, and then she really strikes gold. There's a section called "Management Plan," which lays out, point by point, what the American Diabetes Association recommends. One of these items is a consultation with a registered dietitian familiar with the disease. Marion doesn't remember her doctor mentioning this. Instead, she got a handful of pamphlets and a talk with a nurse practitioner. Should she press for a dietitian? Was the NP fully practiced in this area, or did he just read up before the meeting?

Marion also takes note of the section on referrals, which recommends a visit to an endocrinologist if the treatment plan doesn't control her glucose levels. She didn't get a referral right away, and now she has an idea of when to push for a specialist.

She next notices a section on cardiovascular disease that gives details on what to watch out for. It even has a link to the American Diabetes Association's position statement on aspirin therapy for preventive treatment of heart disease in diabetics. Now Marion is getting information that will allow her to take real control of her condition. She prints the entire set of guidelines, and looks at a few other guidelines before leaving the site.

So far we've considered websites where the information has been condensed and adapted either for popular consumption or use by professionals. Now we will take a quick look at the motherlode of medical information—MedLine. Here you will find abstracts of over nine million journal articles. MedLine is a project of the National Center for Biotechnology Information at the National Library of Medicine, located at the National Institutes of Health. The National Library of Medicine is truly building a monument, as you will see when you start your search. There are many ways to get into MedLine, but probably the best is through MedLinePlus (at www.nlm.nih.gov/medlineplus).

First you will see the familiar consumer-friendly resources. Take some time with these—they may answer your questions. But if you have a specific question that you can't get answered anywhere else, click on "MedLine" or go there directly (through www.ncbi.nlm.

nih.gov/PubMed). If you want a demonstration of how important it is to have a specific query in mind when you approach MedLine, just type in "diabetes." When we tried this, we got 145,985 hits! Even limiting the search to the last thirty days delivered over 400 hits. So only go to MedLine if you know what you are looking for.

Marion remembers reading about a new diabetes drug, Rezulin or troglitazone, that a newspaper claimed caused a number of fatalities. Her doctor mentioned it as a possible treatment. Should she be concerned? MedLine would be the place to get the most recent information. She types in "diabetes AND Rezulin OR troglitazone," and limits her search to the last year. She finds two articles right at the top of her list of 157: "Troglitazone-associated hepatic failure" and "Severe hepatotoxicity associated with troglitazone." Both are less than two months old. She'll need help with the terminology, but she's poised on the leading edge of medical research.

Once you have the citations from MedLine, you need to take an extra step to get the articles. Your librarian might be able to help if you take the full citation, including the volume number and page number, with you. Or you can order the articles from a service like Infotrieve (www.infotrieve.com), which also has a search engine linked to MedLine. You may have to pay over ten dollars for each article, so try your library first.

Most of the time, you won't have to go into medical journal articles to make sure you are getting the best care from your HMO. But when you want to show something to your doctor, you shouldn't give him anything less. Doctors don't make decisions based on newspaper or magazine articles. If you are really serious about changing his mind about your treatment, only material from an established medical journal will do.

Researching a serious condition is an ongoing process, but don't worry. Once you are over the initial fact-gathering, you will find that continuing your education becomes much easier. In cases like Marion's, committed patients usually settle into a rhythm of research that becomes almost habitual. They might subscribe to a magazine, take part in an Internet discussion group, or become a member of a foundation. But either way, they have managed to lift themselves above the HMO madness with information.

STARTING POINTS:
SELECTED GENERAL INFORMATION WEBSITES

MedicineNet: www.medicinenet.com
News, updates, and a searchable medical dictionary. General information on diseases and treatments, procedures and tests, drugs and first aid. Run by "a network of doctors producing comprehensive, up-to-date health information for the public." Bookmark the medical dictionary if you don't have one at home.

AMA Health Insight: www.ama-assn.org/consumer.htm
The consumer section of the American Medical Association's website. Original articles for selected conditions, top medical news, self-assessment quizzes, a medical glossary, and an "ask a doctor" section. The "human atlas" section gives you informative annotated pictures of organs and systems with explanations of different parts.

Drug InfoNet: www.druginfonet.com
Official package inserts and patient package inserts on selected drugs. If you can't find a specific drug on this site, the "manufacturer information" section gives contact information for drug companies.

Mediconsult: www.mediconsult.com
Incredibly easy to use, this site provides and gives educational material, journal articles, conference highlights, news, a glossary, and information on drugs. There's also a gateway to MedLine and help with using this database. Most of the site is free; for a fee (around $200), you can get an online report from a specialist after filling out a form about your condition.

CNN Health: www.cnn.com/health/index.html
As with all health information from news organizations, be sure to check up on any article's claims. That said, this site can give you a well-organized wealth of recent news on many conditions. Look for the "in-depth information" box on the right-hand side, a little more than halfway down the page. Select an illness, and you will be taken to a list of associations, with links. Click on the button above the list, and you get recent CNN stories on the subject.

The Virtual Hospital: www.vh.org
From the University of Iowa College of Medicine. Good educational materials, but sometimes difficult to navigate.

MedHelp International: www.medhelp.org
An excellent nontechnical, selective library, easily accessible through searches. Links to organizations and groups. Consumer forums moderated

STARTING POINTS (continued)

by specialists can answer your questions, and or even help you come up with new questions to ask. A patient-to-patient network can offer support from people who share your concerns. Medical news updated daily.

MedicineNet: www.medicinenet.com
A good glossary, and the "conditions and treatments" section gives drugs related to the illness, procedures and tests, news, related diseases, and frequently asked questions.

HealthFinder: www.healthfinder.gov
Nontechnical articles, organizations, and links from the Department of Health and Human Services. A great place to start.

Mayo Clinic Health Oasis: www.mayohealth.org
Original articles in the "health library," a glossary, and a good search engine. Special "centers" for asthma and allergies, Alzheimer's, cancer, children's health, heart disease, nutrition, and men's and women's health. At the "centers" you can even sign up for e-mail notices to have news delivered electronically.

National Organization of Rare Disorders: www.rarediseases.org
A powerful tool for anyone who has a disease that isn't addressed else-where. The site offers articles, information on local chapters and support groups, and even information on hard-to-find equipment and drugs.

National Guideline Clearinghouse: www.guideline.gov
As detailed in the text, this is a site primarily for professionals, but the careful consumer can gain insight into what their treatment plan might look like.

Agency for Health Care Policy and Research: www.ahcpr.gov
Like the National Guideline Clearinghouse (a project of this agency), you can get guidelines here on selected treatments. See the "Clinical Practice Guidelines Online" in the "Clinical Information" section. Unlike the NGC, these guidelines are sponsored by the AHCPR, which also provides a con-sumer version. It's an ongoing project, so your condition may not yet be listed.

MedLine: www.ncbi.nlm.nih.gov/pubmed
This is the public access point to MedLine, the massive database of jour-nal abstracts from the National Library of Medicine. This is highly techni-cal stuff, so approach MedLine with specific searches in mind, and be sure to get professional help in explaining the articles you find. Full text is not available. You will have to order articles from a service like Infotrieve (www.infotrieve.com) or get help at your library.

I've Done My Research. How Do I Present It to My Doctor?

As you return from your fact-finding expedition, you will feel more in control, assured, and confident about your ability to take part in deciding what treatment is best for you. You will return to your HMO a transformed patient. But now, how can you relay what you have learned to your doctor without stepping on her toes or making her feel like you are questioning her judgment? As you go into consultation with your doctor, you will need to avoid acting like a consumer if you want to maintain the mutual relationship you have built.

Think of the consultation as an extension of your research. Your doctor is a more valuable resource than all the books you have read and all the websites you have visited. She can answer specific questions about how the diagnosed disease affects you. She can look at the data you have gathered and decide how it applies to your case. Remember that the consultation is all about you. It's not about the merits and faults of a recent study, and definitely not about the boy in Washington who had the same condition but was saved by a pioneering treatment. The study and the story *might* have applications to your case, and that's what your doctor can help you decide.

Remember to read your doctor. Try to get a sense of how open she is to your research. If she seems resistant, approach the topic carefully. It's always a good idea to bring up your findings with a question. These can usually start with the phrase "What do you think of . . ." Make it clear that while you pursue your research, her input remains paramount.

There's a good chance that your doctor will be pleased that you are learning about your condition. It says to her that you are ready to look at your problem objectively, the same way she is. This side-by-side objective view is a cornerstone of a mutual relationship. But just to be sure no egos are injured and no additional problems created, follow these tips for bringing research to your doctor:

- Don't launch into what you know as soon as you walk into the room. Each follow-up visit should still involve HEAD to some degree, perhaps with less emphasis on past history and more emphasis on any changes in your condition. The time to bring up your research is at "D"—the decision.

- Bring copies of relevant articles, but not more than a few. These articles should be from high-level sources. Journal articles are the best. Fact sheets and guidelines from organizations are good. Avoid bringing in newspaper clippings or e-mail messages from someone in your Internet discussion group. Even if your doctor reads these, he will just have to do research of his own to verify it in a journal or manual. If you really want him to consider your information, save him this extra step.

- Avoid the life-saving anecdote. If it's just one case, it doesn't mean anything to your doctor. His scientific gold standard is the double-blind placebo-controlled trial. The treatment that saved someone's life may have killed someone else. To doctors, anecdotes are just gossip and mostly a waste of time.

- Avoid using the words "experimental" when talking about treatments. For one thing, if it's experimental, your HMO probably won't approve it. For another, the word means different things in different contexts. Many cancer treatments are called "experimental" because they are currently being evaluated in clinical trials, but since we are still figuring out how cancer works, these treatments can also be the standard of care.

- Bring it all back to the plan. How might this research being done in Boston affect our plan? I read that this illness puts me at risk for heart disease. How does that affect our plan?

- Always let your doctor know that you value her opinion. In the end, you will decide for yourself, but her contribution is critical.

You have done your research in order to protect yourself against the cost-cutting measures of your HMO, but you shouldn't have to protect yourself against your doctor. Most doctors will be excited to be treating a patient who shows up informed and ready to make the right decision. By being a patient who is both objective and concerned, you can trigger your doctor's problem-solving instincts, reminding her that her job can be rewarding, even in the shadow of the HMO. You have your doctor's attention. It's time to work on building a team.

How Do I Build a Team?

Good doctors never take on serious conditions or procedures alone. The more serious the condition, the more different parts of the body are affected. That means specialists have to get involved. Unlike private practice doctors in the old system who relied on a loose network for referrals, HMOs have great team-building potential. A good HMO should have all manner of services, from the highly trained specialist to the non-MD consultant. The challenge for you is to pull these resources together and get them to focus on you.

The resources are there, but you can't count on any one doctor to coordinate the entire treatment. HMOs are too large, and their doctors too busy, to manage every aspect of your treatment. You will have to be the manager, quarterback, and sometimes coach of your medical team. If you get a referral to a new specialist, don't think of it as an assignment. Think of it as a recruiting opportunity. Let that specialist know that he is part of something larger than this one visit.

"If you want to build a ship," wrote Antoine de Saint-Exupéry, "don't try rallying people to get the wood, distribute the tasks and organize the work, rather inspire people with the desire for the wide ocean." Don't let your team members focus only on their small part of the treatment. Don't tell them that you are there just because Dr. Primary sent you. Let them know your wider goals, that you are trying to regain your health or prevent certain complications. Let them know what else is going on. Then let them do their part.

As Marion performed her research, she kept track of different parts of her body that are affected by diabetes. She then created specific health goals for each. Once she can express these goals clearly, she can make a list of the professionals she wants on her team. She knows from the guidelines she read that her blood sugar should be at a certain level to prevent damage to her eyes, kidneys, and nervous system. Who can help her reach this goal? Her primary care physician is ready to help, so she assigns him to this area. She knows that if complications arise, she should add an endocrinologist to her team. She knows that one important way to keep her blood sugar down is through drugs. That means that her pharmacist should be drafted as well.

Don't think of your pharmacist as a clerk behind the counter. He's been trained in much more than pulling containers off the shelf. He may be even more up-to-date on new drugs and their effects than your doctor. Think of him as a drug specialist. Ask him questions about side effects, dosages, and possible interactions, even if you've already talked to your doctor about this. Let him know about your condition, and get him on your team.

Marion's research told her that she should watch her diet, and the guidelines she read told her that she should get help from a dietician trained in diabetes treatment. Is there someone like this on her health plan? It could be a nutritionist or a nurse practitioner, as long as they have been trained in diabetes management. Marion will find out because she knows it's important. She can read up on her recommended diet, but she still has to have that individualized attention.

Marion also learned that she should watch out for foot ulcers. People with diabetes can lose sensation in their extremities, and so a wound on the foot can go unnoticed. This can lead to an amputation if not caught early. She needs a podiatrist on her team. At first, it will be just for a consultation, but if anything goes wrong, she will want to know that a podiatrist is already in her corner.

In the same way, moving from her knowledge about the disease to defining a goal, Marion adds an ophthalmologist and cardiologist to her team. She realizes that she may add other team members after talking to her doctor and nurse practitioner. That reminds her—the nurse practitioner should definitely be recruited.

The nurse practitioner is playing an increasingly important role in the HMO medical team, and she is a great choice. While doctors may be inclined to err on the side of their own independence, being a team player is what nursing is all about. Your nurse practitioner knows HEAD, so you can talk to her in that language. She knows about specialists. In fact, studies have revealed that NPs are more likely to refer to a specialist than primary care doctors. She knows about drugs and their interactions. And she has more time to spend with you than your doctor. Don't think of your nurse practitioner as your doctor's assistant. She's your second-string quarterback, ready to step in when you can't make the play yourself. She is especially important if you must undergo high-tech treatments like transplants, unusual surgeries, and other treatments for extremely debilitating conditions.

Once Marion has settled on the team members from her HMO,

she begins to think about team members from outside the HMO. She intends to see an endocrinologist outside the plan for an information-only consultation. He's on her list. She plans to contact the American Diabetes Association to see what resources they can offer. She's seen an acupuncturist for years for her lower back pain. He might not be able to help, but it won't hurt to ask him about diabetes treatment. Marion even goes to her church to inquire about the diabetes support group that meets on Thursdays. Now that all the pieces of the puzzle are in place, Marion is ready to put her team to work.

As team leader, Marion knows that she will have to coordinate her players. She will bring records with her, keep track of treatments, prescriptions, procedures, and results. She starts a diabetes diary for this information and also uses it to monitor her exercise program, diet, and glucose levels. She brings this diary to every appointment, and gives each player a glimpse of the wide ocean—her general health.

What Have I Accomplished?

By keeping yourself informed, you will know what you need. You know why you want to see a specialist, and you know why it's important. You have the tools to convince your doctor that the treatment is necessary, and you've won him over to your side. He'll be ready to be your partner, advocate, and team member. You can look at your HMO's plan for treatment closely, and be ready to analyze it for dangerous money-saving shortcuts. Your protection, power, and potential for health have all grown in the light of your research.

As you probably suspect, HMOs love to say no. But by doing your research, keeping a complete record of what you have learned, and putting together a treatment plan, you have taken a preemptive step against their refusals. In the next chapter, we will show you how to use your research to appeal denied treatment. With your doctor on your side and the knowledge you have gained, you can make it virtually impossible for your HMO to turn you down.

~ 7 ~

Days of Denial

Getting through Your Appeal

> **QUESTIONS THIS CHAPTER ANSWERS**
> - *Why was my treatment denied?*
> - *What does "medically necessary" mean?*
> - *How do I make an appeal?*
> - *Where can I get help?*
> - *When should I leave my health plan?*
> - *How do I choose a new health plan?*

A doctor we know in Los Angeles told us about a time she treated a patient—let's call him Drake—for throat cancer. Drake had flown in from Albuquerque, and his local HMO had agreed to cover the out-of-network treatment—a surgery that this doctor was well known for. But before the operation, Drake developed pneumonia, and the operation had to be rescheduled.

The doctor called the patient's HMO and explained that she wanted to minimize her patient's suffering by keeping him in the hospital for a few days to treat his lungs before performing surgery on his throat. The answer she got was swift and shocking: the HMO would still cover the operation, but declined to cover the hospital stay for pneumonia. They wanted him to fly back to New Mexico, with a fever and water in his lungs, to be treated there. Then they would fly him back to L.A. again for the operation.

The doctor was outraged: "The company's decision was medically inappropriate—completely inappropriate. How could they let him go back when there was a cancer growing in his throat?" Yes, the decision was completely inappropriate medically. But the HMO's motivation was clear. They had already paid their capitated network doctors about $25 per month to treat his pneumonia. If he stayed in the L.A. hospital, they would have to fork over about $1,000 per day. If they allowed many patients to do this, they would go bankrupt.

HMOs make money when they deny care. If they didn't deny care, they would cease to exist. But that doesn't mean you can't get the care you need. Even the stingiest HMO has to follow its own rules. HMOs *have* to provide care if it is "medically necessary."

When the L.A. surgeon broke the bad news to Drake, she could hear the concern in his voice. He immediately started asking questions about his pneumonia. How bad is it? Can I actually fly home without making it worse? These questions opened the surgeon's eyes to her patient's condition. She wasn't used to treating pneumonia, and hadn't asked these questions herself. She flashed back to her conversation with the Albuquerque HMO. "I want to minimize this patient's suffering," she had told them. "He wants to stay here to get over his pneumonia." She didn't frame her plan in terms of a medical necessity—only in terms of her wishes and her patient's.

The patient's fever was higher than the day before. He was delirious. He was having trouble breathing. He was in an emergency. And his plan *had* to cover nonnetwork emergency care. The doctor realized that she hadn't expressed this fully to the HMO. They didn't have a complete clinical picture. She placed a second call, and had the patient's chart faxed to the Albuquerque medical director. Now the case was clear, and the HMO, by its own contract, couldn't deny coverage for the patient's pneumonia. Thanks to the new approach, this story had a happy ending.

The guidelines we have given you so far—using HEAD, developing a preventive plan, doing your homework—should keep you from ever having to fight through an appeal. You know how to give your doctor a complete clinical picture. You know how to keep yourself from getting sick, and how to catch problems at an early stage. You know how to research your condition to back up your claim.

But Murphy's Law still applies. You may be denied perfectly appropriate and necessary medical care because of a bureaucratic tangle. You may have a treatment rubber-stamped "No way" by a utilization review doctor just because he had a bad lunch. You may be caught up in an organization-wide cost-cutting campaign that has nothing to do with you. If you've followed our advice so far, you should be getting along famously with your health plan. But you still have to prepare yourself for "no."

One might ask, "How can members of HMOs' utilization review committees denying payment for case after case actually sleep at night?" The answer is really quite simple. The reviewers don't see patients, only numbers, statistics, and reports. Steps are taken to ensure that no emotional commitment can "interfere" with their business decisions. The HMO review committee members judge the validity of dozens of claims on a daily basis, claims that are nothing more than a piece of paper or a spreadsheet. Providing as much information as possible to the review board is a crucial component to getting the care you deserve. But what happens if your request is rejected?

In this chapter, we will show you how to use what you have learned so far to turn a "no" into a "yes." HEAD will help, your preventive risk-analysis will come into play, and the research you have done will prove invaluable. And you will learn the two most important words for an HMO patient: "Medically necessary."

What Is "Medically Necessary?"

The strange thing about this term is that no one used it before managed care came along. When indemnity insurance was paying the bills, we got all the care that was necessary and quite a bit of care that was unnecessary. No one was asking questions.

When HMOs started taking over and attempting to keep costs down, they invented the term "medically necessary" as a way to deny all the care they could get away with. If you look at your explanation of benefits, you are sure to find this phrase. They are only two words, but they have incredible power. Everyone uses the phrase, everyone wants to define it. A debate in Congress continues as this book goes to press between doctors and insurers over who should decide what is medically necessary. Both sides know what is at stake—power over billions of dollars in health services.

Let's take a look at a typical use of the phrase. As one contract puts it, medical services are covered "only if in the judgment of a Plan Physician, they are medically necessary to prevent, diagnose, or treat a medical condition. A service or item is medically necessary only if a Plan Physician determines that its *omission* would directly affect a Member's health" (emphasis ours).

Pay attention to how this wording sets you up for denials. The HMO is *not* asking "Will this treatment make the patient better?" The contract asks "Will denying this treatment make the patient worse?" The whole idea is to provide the bare minimum. That's how managed care saves money.

If you keep this in mind, you will already have learned something crucial about how to appeal. Never say that the treatment will make you better. Always emphasize that *not* getting the treatment will make you worse, perhaps so much worse that you will require more expensive care. Now you are using the HMO's own logic. It may be a strange way to think, but it's the only way to get your point across.

If you think that's strange, read the above excerpt again; there's another example of HMO logic hidden in the phrasing. What is medically necessary? It doesn't say. All the contract says is that a Plan Physician decides. So a treatment is medically necessary if, and only if, it's "medically necessary." Welcome to managed care's hall of mirrors. By being vague, the HMO seeks to retain complete control. But if you know how to work the system, you can wrest control away for yourself.

You can break out of this circular logic. You can use this tool that managed care has created. "Medical necessity" is a loose, undefined, fuzzy term. It always will be that way. It's not a standard or a yardstick, even if it looks like one. That means you can adopt it for yourself and your health.

There's an old joke about three umpires discussing their chosen profession. The first one says, "There are balls and strikes, and it's my job to call them." The second one says, "Sure, there are balls, and then there are strikes, but I call them like I see them." The third one, much older and wiser, says, "There are balls and there are strikes, but they aren't *anything* until I call them." Medical necessity isn't defined. It isn't anything until someone calls it. If you pay close attention to your condition and work the appeals process the right way, you can be the one who makes the call.

What Is the Goal of My Appeal?

When you are denied care that you believe you need and are entitled to, of course you may think that you are just being screwed. The typical reaction is to fight to win. That's how we have been trained as consumers. If we get shoddy merchandise or bad service, our appeals are driven by the idea that we can and should win. But while it's easy to spot a broken television or a shoddy repair job, it's incredibly hard to define when our health is at stake. Our bodies are far more complicated than televisions, and medical science doesn't always have clear-cut answers. In the health care arena, our goals should be slightly adjusted.

The goal of your appeal should be to get the best care. It should *not* be simply to win. It should *not* be to force the HMO into giving you what you *think* you need. Approach the appeals process as an extension of your research. Always ask yourself, "What is really best for me?" Don't just call it like you see it. Leave the question open until you are ready to make the call.

Dr. Feinberg is knee-deep in appeals. It's his job to review appealed cases with his colleagues and make the tough choices. Luckily for both his group's patients and his group, he is committed to finding ways to provide excellent patient care and save money at the same time. This requires a bit more brains and effort than many doctors in his position are capable of. Denial of a claim is always the easiest route: The exam wasn't complete? Tell the patient no. The paperwork is a mess? Just tell the patient no. The patient wants to go outside the network for advanced treatment? Forget it. It's too much trouble to do the exam again, fix the paperwork, or look into the advanced treatment that might actually save the plan money. It's always easier to say no, and too many denials happen just because someone was lazy.

But once you get someone to actually focus on you, surprising things can happen. If a medical director really looks at the case, it's like getting an automatic second opinion. This is where HMOs can really shine. You might not get the treatment you asked for, but you might get something better.

Before Dr. Feinberg came to his present position, he once sat on an appeals board that was considering an appeal for continuance of psychiatric care. The patient in question was close to using up his allotted visits, and both he and the psychiatrist felt that the treatment should continue. The patient felt great about his treatment and his doctor, and was asking for more. The question was, as always, "What is medically necessary in this case?"

When the board looked at the case, they saw a total mess. It was clear to everyone in the room that the patient had a treatable mental disorder that the doctor had not even diagnosed. As a result, the doctor was treating his patient improperly, both in his choice of therapy and in his choice of medications. The patient and doctor had a great relationship, and a great deal of trust, but the patient wasn't getting the appropriate care. In fact, he was getting worse.

If the HMO hadn't limited the number of visits, no one would have ever discovered how bad things had gotten. If the psychiatrist had been seeing the patient on a fee-for-service basis, there would have been no check or balance on his poor decisions. But here the patient got a room full of experienced doctors to discuss his case and plan a better course. Forget second opinions. When managed care works well, you can get a swarm of opinions.

In this case, the patient didn't exactly "win" his appeal, but he wasn't denied either. The appeals board just changed the plan. They limited the number of visits, but the patient was allowed to continue with his doctor. The committee resolved to monitor the situation. If it didn't improve, they planned to begin a transition to a more appropriate therapist. Either the care would improve, or the patient would be moved to a better situation. Either way, the patient wins, even if not necessarily in the way he expected.

That's the way it *should* work. But we're not writing this book with our heads in the sand. We know that laziness, incompetence, and just plain apathy rule the day in many HMOs. That shouldn't change your goal. You want to get better, not beat the system. As you wade into the appeals process, your patience is likely to be tried, too much of your time consumed, and you may feel like you will never win. Maybe you won't, but that's not your goal. Your goal is to get better. You can use all the resources HMOs put into the appeals process to help you figure out exactly *how* you can get better. Again, an appeal is a chance to improve, extend, and direct your research.

As it was with your ten-minute office visit and your research, staying organized will pave the way to a happy conclusion. Asking the right questions at the right time will get you the right answers. If you ever hear the word "no" from your HMO, the first question you should ask is "Why was my treatment denied?"

Why Was My Treatment Denied?

Money. Your treatment was denied because of money. It's not because no one cares, and it's not because they can't help you. In HMOs, "No way" means "We won't pay." It's the only way they can keep their business afloat. It's necessary to close the gates on as many procedures as possible. HMOs will argue that they never really deny *care*, they just deny paying for it. "Patients," they say, "can always see whomever they wish, at any time, as long as they pay the bills." But you pay your medical insurance premiums. Don't you get a say?

How can you possibly get an appeal through an HMO when it's all about money? The procedure you want will cost, so isn't your care completely incompatible with the plan's balance sheet? Not quite. Remember that you are in a huge gray area between big business and charity. Managed care isn't like normal business—in an HMO money doesn't talk. It whispers.

No HMO will come right out and say that you are being denied because of money, but it's always true. An HMO that did admit this would be a malpractice lawyer's ultimate fantasy. You wouldn't even have to have a law degree to sway a jury against an HMO that admitted what everyone knows is true—that it's all about money. And so almost every denial is based on this notion of "medical necessity."

The plan is not usually going to give you detailed reasons for your denial. It doesn't have to, and administrators know that providing full documentation up front just creates a paper trail that a lawyer might follow later. "Not medically necessary" is usually all they have to say. That creates confusion and frustration among patients more than anything else. No other practice is surer to make you feel like the HMO is a cold, impenetrable monolith. It's your job to figure out why you were denied.

Dig a little deeper. There are reasons for HMOs to summon up the "medically necessary" phantasm. If your condition *is* a medical necessity and you were denied anyway, it means something went wrong. It could be a problem with paperwork. It could have happened in the examining room. Or it could be due to general pressure across the organization to cut back on the care you need. And of course, you may find that you were denied because your procedure really isn't needed.

If you really do need the procedure, the denial has little to do with your condition and everything to do with perception. Someone in the appeals ladder just doesn't see things the same way you do. It's your job to make them see the same problem the same way, or find a third way that satisfies their definition of "medical necessity" and yours. Always remember that a ball can look like a strike if you tilt the umpire's head a little to the side.

Denial by Clerical Error, Part One: Medical Record Mistakes

You've done everything right. You used HEAD during your office visit, and you've done your research. You and your doctor know exactly what has to happen next. You are both surprised when your treatment is refused. After all, the HMO's own guidelines provide for exactly what you and your doctor want.

Sometimes you can be denied just because someone didn't cross their Ts. Some piece of information was available, but it didn't get through to the review upstairs. It's a simple clerical error, and in these huge organizations that shuffle tens of thousands of papers a day, it's a common problem. Say you are being treated for asthma. You and your doctor have tracked your treatment, and you aren't getting better. By the HMO's own guidelines, after three failed treatments you should get a nebulizer. But you were refused.

What happened? Someone in the review process punched in "2" on a form when he should have punched in "3." Someone didn't see the description of your last failed treatment. Your doctor's handwriting was so bad someone couldn't make it out. These are the real reasons you got a denial, but all the HMO says is that "it's not medically necessary."

What to do:
- Get a copy of your medical records. You have every right to see them.
- Get a copy of the HMO's treatment guidelines for your condition.
- See if you can get a copy of the HMO's denial in writing.

- See if your doctor will write down his version of events.
- Call the review number and explain that you think there has been a mistake. Describe your condition, and quote the relevant guidelines, giving the page number in the managed care contract.
- If that doesn't work, write a letter to the medical director. We'll talk about that letter later in this chapter.

Most of the time, this should be all it takes. Once someone with power has the complete information, everything should go your way. When you get a denial for a commonplace treatment that both you and your doctor know you should have, stay calm. Look for an administrative error first. It might be just that simple.

Denial by Clerical Error, Part Two: Accounting Mistakes

Paperwork errors occur just as frequently in financial record keeping as in medical record keeping. This is especially true whenever you are seeking out-of-network care—a process that creates a whirlwind of paperwork in the HMO accountant's office. All sorts of things can go wrong. Your prescription costs or allotted visits may have been miscalculated, incorrectly putting you over a certain limit. The HMO may have "forgotten" that you have already paid your deductible. Since this fight is with bookkeepers rather than with doctors and nurses, you may encounter belligerence and rudeness. These detail-oriented people hate to admit mistakes. If you manage to keep a cooler head, you will prevail.

Bookkeeping errors can lead to some ridiculous situations. Dr. Theodosakis once fell victim to this kind of absurdity. Suffering from a thyroid condition, he knew exactly what tests he needed and where to get them—in this case, out of the network. That shouldn't have been a problem. His PPO allowed self-referrals to out-of-network doctors for a co-payment of 20 percent. So knowing that his plan would cover 80 percent of the fee, he went ahead and got the tests.

But when it came time for his plan to make good on their promise, they refused. The plan simply claimed that his tests weren't covered. They were wrong. Dr. Theodosakis knew that they owed his specialist 80 percent of his fee. Dr. Theodosakis began the appeals process, which went on for months. He became increasingly curious. How far would this go?

Finally, his case was ready to go to the appeals board, involving a face-to-face meeting between Dr. Theodosakis and the HMO review committee. Just before this was about to happen, however, someone from the plan called and admitted that a mistake had been made. Accounting had sent the bill through asking for *full* payment. So of course it was denied. But since the plan hadn't spelled out its reasons, Dr. Theodosakis thought they were declining to pay their 80 percent. They were actually declining to pay 100 percent. So the whole battle was, in the end, over nothing.

What to do:

- Keep your own records. Anticipate that there will, someday, be an accounting error. Keep track of how much you pay and how much your HMO pays. Keep track of exact dates, and who provided the care.

- Always request copies of bills. Hold onto those copies.

- Be aware of caps on your prescriptions and visits. Don't wait until your benefit runs out before you start asking questions.

- Make sure you and your HMO know what the disagreement is. As with the example of Dr. Theodosakis's thyroid problem, you may be fighting over nothing.

- Try to bypass the normal appeals process and go directly to accounting.

- Avoid getting your doctor involved in a fight that's only about money. Keep him appraised of what's going on, especially if the HMO owes him, but fight the battle yourself. You want your relationship to be about care, not about dollars.

Denials due to paperwork errors can be incredibly frustrating. But the fact that they are so common should tell you something: keep your own records. The information in your HMO's file should be an accurate, comprehensive account of the state of your health and how it's paid for. Sometimes, clerical errors will make it fall short. You should always be ready to point out exactly where your file and the truth part ways. Then an appeal can become a simple process of getting your file back on track.

Denial by Examining-Room Error

You and your doctor have done your paperwork perfectly. All the right boxes are checked, all the available evidence has been entered into your chart. Still, your treatment has been denied as not medically necessary. What went wrong?

Sometimes care that's perfectly appropriate and necessary can be denied because something was left out of the exam or history. The paperwork may be in order, but the reviewers don't have a complete clinical picture. If you used HEAD during your visit, you will probably be confident that you gave your doctor all the information he needs. But if you get a denial, it's time to think about what you might have left out.

It could also be your doctor's mistake. Maybe he didn't do an appropriately thorough exam. Say you complained about a pain in your side, and your doctor didn't check for a swollen liver. If he writes "patient reports abdominal pain," and puts you on a course to treat jaundice, the HMO is likely to reject this treatment as not medically necessary. It is right to do so. Your doctor needs to check for a distended liver.

We see this happen all the time with headaches. The doctor is faced with a suffering patient who is worried about brain tumors. The doctor should do a complete neurological exam, which includes testing the patient's speech patterns, vision, and ability to make spatial relations. But these exams take time, so some doctors might just send the patient off for an MRI. These scans are one of the most frequently denied tests in HMOs, partly because they were so overused before managed care came along, partly because they are so expensive. So if a utilization review doctor sees an MRI request, he is very likely to reject it unless the primary care physician or neurologist has documented findings in your exam to justify this expensive imaging test.

There's a good reason for this. You shouldn't get any treatment or test until all the evidence needed to justify it has been gathered. The problem for you is that the denial won't say what's missing. The HMO doesn't want to give you a roadmap to getting your MRI; that might lead to patients faking symptoms to get expensive tests. So you are left to figure out if you really need what you have been denied.

What to do:

- Review HEAD on your own. Think hard about what you might have left out of the history. Then think about whether the doctor looked for *objective* signs of your symptoms. Did he really look at you?

- Get your medical records. If all the doctor has written is "patient reports," that's a good sign that you need a more complete exam.

- Get back into the examining room if you find that you or your doctor missed a step. When you are there, remember your goal: to paint a complete clinical picture. You are looking for the truth, not just looking to win. You don't want that test or treatment unless you really need it.

- Follow the prescribed course. If the HMO has overruled your own doctor's plan and replaced it with its own, follow the course. But pay close attention to your symptoms. Are they getting worse, better, or staying the same? Keep your primary care physician up to date on your condition as you follow the course.

- Do your research. Focus on your HMO's own guidelines and general reference books for the layperson. Try to figure out what your symptoms might be telling you.

If your doctor makes a mistake that leads to a denial, don't automatically assume that he's incompetent. Many doctors are still getting used to working with managed care. He might not know all the hoops he has to jump through to deliver the treatment you need. He might not be completely familiar with your HMO's guidelines for specific illnesses. He may have contracts with several HMOs, each with its own procedures, hoops, and guidelines. Just because he didn't get it right the first time doesn't mean he's done a bad job.

If a procedure he recommended is refused, he's probably just as upset about it as you are. Doctors absolutely hate having their judgment overruled by someone who hasn't even seen the patient. He will be ready to work with you on your appeal, if it comes to that. But first, you will want to make him understand that both of you should take a second look at the problem to find out what is medically necessary. Then, using HEAD, give him something new to think about.

Denial by Statistic

Meet the utilization review doctor. He's got the thankless job of trying to figure out how to save your HMO even more money. He does this by compiling and analyzing statistics on procedures and their results. If his HMO is above the national average for managed care plan approvals of a given procedure, the plan's doctors are told to avoid overutilization of that procedure. Doctors who get these notices hate the UR doctor's guts.

Lets say Dr. Cruncher, who works for the Health Harvest HMO as a UR doctor, notices that hospitalizations in his organization are above the national average for managed care. His job is to figure out why. He looks at all of Health Harvest's doctors for their hospitalization rates. Dr. DoRight, he finds, is way over the national average. He's sending too many patients to the hospital. A memo goes out to all of Health Harvest's doctors telling them to watch for ways to keep admissions down. Dr. DoRight gets a special note along with this memo, giving him the statistics that Dr. Cruncher has compiled and warning him strongly to avoid "medically unnecessary" hospitalizations.

Dr. Cruncher doesn't know that Dr. DoRight's admission rates are high because his office is situated between a retirement village and a tenement neighborhood where there was a recent tuberculosis outbreak. He doesn't know that Dr. DoRight just got a similar memo for referrals to orthopedic surgeons. Dr. Cruncher doesn't look at the specifics of each case to see if hospitalization was justified or not. The numbers are just too high, and they have to come down.

Dr. DoRight gets this memo on his way in to see you for a persistent cough. You have all the signs of TB. You should be in a hospital. Dr. DoRight knows this, but also knows that he can be deselected at any time, for any reason. He feels like he's on the edge. But here's a patient who needs help. The ethical dilemma is resolved when you wonder out loud if you should be in the hospital. Dr. DoRight writes "patient requests hospitalization" on your chart. There. Now Health Harvest can't blame him for this referral.

When it goes up for review, another UR doctor looks at the chart and only skims the history and exam results. His eyes rest on the words "patient requests." He ponders why the doctor didn't put down his own recommendation, but only for a split second. REQUEST DENIED. This chain of events all started with a batch of statistics, and now you are a statistic as well.

This use of statistics looks suspiciously like "rationed care"—that socialist evil we thought we dodged when we rejected national health insurance. But HMOs aren't supposed to ration care. An HMO will never say you were denied because of organization-wide pressure to keep the averages on a treatment low. But reviewers will apply increased scrutiny and newly tailored guidelines to deny treatments that have been "redlined."

The only way to fight this is to match the number-crunchers' diligence with your own. Then work to bring it all back to you—your condition, your needs, your treatment, your medical necessity. Statistics can't tell anyone whether you should get your treatment or not. But you and your doctor can.

What to do:

- Get the denial in writing, and demand that the reasons for denial be listed. Examine the document for arguments that stretch the boundaries of reason. The rationale for the denial should make sense to you. If it doesn't, you have grounds for appeal.

- Ask your doctor what she thinks. You are more likely to get a straight answer if you avoid directly mentioning the appeal, and focus on what she thinks is the *best* treatment.

- Do your research. Many HMOs will release statistics like the ones that Dr. Cruncher compiled. Compare these to the national averages. If your HMO's numbers are comparable, you can phrase your appeal in this light: "I can see that you allow many patients to get this treatment. What is different about my case?"

- Get second opinions. Go out of the network and pay out of your own pocket if you have to. Most HMOs aren't contractually obliged to listen to outside opinions, but they can still carry weight.

- Get guidelines for treatment from nonnetwork sources. The National Guideline Clearinghouse, discussed in the last chapter, is a great place to start. Seek a professional interpretation, and use it to prove medical necessity.

- Monitor your condition. Any signs that your condition is getting worse, no matter how small, can help your appeal. Remember that most HMO contracts can't omit treatment if that omission will make you worse. Any new symptoms can help clarify exactly what is medically necessary. Act on these new symptoms quickly.

If you find that your denial may be linked to your HMO's use of statistics, you will have them in a corner. HMOs are supposed to manage care, not ration care. No health plan wants to be accused of cold-hearted indifference toward the lives it covers, so any hint that its inner workings might be exposed will get you a quick resolution. The plan's administrators don't want your managed care nightmare to become their public relations nightmare.

Denial by Design: Lack of Coverage

What is covered? What is your benefit? You would think that this question would be spelled out exactly in your contract with your health plan, but that's not always the case. If you look at your contract, or get a copy of your employer's contract with your HMO, you will notice two things. First, it's huge and impenetrable. Second, it's extremely vague. While some treatments and procedures are spelled out in detail, others are left to the whim of the reviewers. Here again, it will come back to medical necessity.

We hear about denials based on lack of coverage most frequently when the denied treatment is deemed "experimental" or "investigative." Managed care plans keep an ever-changing list of approved procedures. When a new procedure or drug comes to light, UR doctors comb reports and journal articles to help the HMO decide if it should be added to the list. If they find that the procedure is described as "experimental," or if they decide the clinical study didn't include enough participants, they will recommend that the procedure or drug should *not* be covered. Most of the time, covered treatments must have a substantial amount of evidence from multiple studies to show that they work and are cost-effective. The treatments covered by an HMO are rarely on the cutting edge of medicine.

If a treatment has been called "experimental," that doesn't mean that the treatment isn't medically appropriate, but it does mean that the HMO's reviewers can say that it's not medically necessary. They will say that there's no proof that denying the treatment will make your condition worse. In cases like this, you may feel helpless to fight your health plan. They've got the "proof," the studies, and the statistics. Unless you are a trained specialist, you will find it difficult to argue your case on the facts.

If you decide to push for coverage of an "experimental" treatment, you will need the help of an out-of-network specialist. If your condition is life-threatening, you may need the help of a lawyer. You will need to move your research into high gear. Battles over "experimental" procedures can be long and involved, and there's no guarantee you will win. The HMO wrote the contract, and it has anticipated your every move.

But there is another way. If an HMO's reviewers won't listen to your medical arguments, they might listen to your financial arguments. If you can arrange for the "experimental" treatment to be cheaper for your HMO, you will take the teeth out of their denial. Dr. Theodosakis pulled this off when he needed surgery on his elbow during his medical training.

Dr. Theodosakis was covered for an invasive surgery that would require cutting open the joint to solve the problem. The treatment would also require months of physical therapy to get his elbow back to normal. But he knew of a surgeon who was pioneering a new arthroscopic technique, where the surgery could be performed with a few simple incisions and advanced equipment. With this procedure, Dr. Theodosakis would require only minimal physical therapy to complete the treatment. But the plan wouldn't cover this "new surgery."

While Dr. Theodosakis worked on explaining to his plan that this procedure was better for both him and them in the long run, he negotiated a price with the out-of-network specialist. His goal was to get the price of the arthoscopy down while getting his plan to pay more of the bill. All along, he realized that he might have to make up the difference between what his surgeon would charge and what his plan would pay. But he also knew that he'd rather take some money out of his own pocket than expose himself to the risks of the traditional, more invasive surgery.

In the end, the surgeon's price and his plan's coverage matched almost exactly. Everyone emerged a winner. The surgeon got business he wouldn't otherwise have had. Dr. Theodosakis's HMO avoided the risks associated with the more invasive surgery. And Dr. Theodosakis got the best treatment available.

Patients haven't yet gotten used to the idea of negotiating for treatment, but managed care has rewritten the rules, and now it's a necessity. Non-HMO doctors, the ones who often provide the best treatments and pioneer the newest procedures, are realizing that they have to be flexible with their rates if they want to treat patients. They won't mind a friendly negotiation. Many of them will even advocate for you by writing letters to your plan, explaining the procedure and the cost-saving benefits. They want the business just as much as you want the treatment.

What to do:

- Get the figures. Find out what your HMO's treatment will cost, including all follow-up visits, drugs, and therapy. Compare that to what your preferred treatment will cost.

- Don't be afraid to negotiate. Work both sides—your HMO and the out-of-network doctor—at the same time.

- Get your primary care doctor on your side. She will be excited about the potential of new procedures. Doctors just love this sort of thing.

- Get the nonnetwork doctor on your side. Explain that you want the procedure, but you are having trouble getting your HMO to pay. He will understand.

- Be ready to pay out of pocket for some part of the procedure. If you do pay, you just might be able to convince your HMO to reimburse you. If the procedure was a success, report back to the plan on how well it worked. There's always a chance the plan's administrators will see how you and they have benefited at the same time.

- Get the care you need. Don't let a long appeals process make your condition worse. Your health is more important than the money you may have to pay.

We have covered the most common and most general reasons that treatments are denied—clerical error, medical error, money-saving strategies, and lack of coverage. Your denial may be due to several of these problems at the same time, and you will have to develop an individual strategy that accounts for all of these possibilities. But just by asking the question, "Why was my claim denied?" you can move beyond the vague logic HMOs use to deny care. By getting to the root of the problem, you can shift the debate over "medical necessity" to more solid ground.

Next, we will discuss the two most important steps in the appeals process: the phone call and the appeal letter. Once you know why claims are denied, your conversations and correspondence can address specific problems and get specific results.

How Do I Place an Appeals Call?

The first stop for an appeal is usually with the HMO's toll-free number. It might be called the customer service hotline or the information hotline, but every HMO has one. The problem is, all sorts of calls will come into this number, so you will have to be specific about what you want.

You are making an appeal, *not* a complaint or grievance. A complaint is over poor service—the doctor was rude, the pharmacist didn't honor your prescription, you were charged too much. An appeal is an attempt to change a medical decision that affects your health. Be very, very clear on this point. Many needless delays are caused by patients who fail to make this distinction from the beginning.

It's especially important to keep this in mind if your HMO has outsourced appeals management. As HMOs attempt to recommit to quality, the appeals process has only become more complicated. An HMO might take appeals away from a medical group and handle it itself. It might carve it out completely and give it to a third party. You may have to appeal to a different entity for drug-related appeals than you do for procedure-related appeals. In short, you may get the runaround.

The person on the other end of the line may have little sympathy with your situation. He may not have complete information on the appeals process, the HMO benefits, or other questions you may have. He is not going to put you at ease or take care of things for you. Most of the time, he is far from being a doctor. He probably isn't even a nurse. His job is to just fill out a form. All you can do at this stage is give complete information and not take out your frustrations or blame him. Remember, the operator had nothing to do with your predicament.

Every appeal will be different, and every HMO will have different procedures for your appeal. But the phone call is usually the first step, and there are several general guidelines you should follow to make sure you are off to a good start.

- Be prepared. You should have your member ID number ready, as well as your social security number, and, if you have one, your medical group number. Member lists are being merged and broken down all the time. The more you can tell the operator about yourself the better.

- Don't place this call when you are rushed or at work. You will be placed on hold, sent through voice mail, and may be given other numbers to call. Set aside some time for this important first step.

- Get the operator's name. Do this when you start the conversation, and write it down. Call the operator by name during your conversation. If you treat the operator like a real person, he will do the same.

- See if you can get a copy of your denial in writing. HMOs tend to convey bad news verbally through your doctor. Get the paperwork sent to you.

- Use HEAD to describe yourself and your conditions. Give the relevant symptoms and history. Sure, this information should be in your chart, but you can't be too certain.

- Be sure you give your exact diagnosis when you call. The person on the phone might not know what you are talking about, but the review nurse or UR doctor will.

- Give the exact treatment you were prescribed, and the exact treatment you want, in medical terminology. Again, even though you aren't talking to a doctor, a medical professional will, at some point, look at the form the operator has filled out.

- Get a response time. Be clear about when you should expect to hear back.

Keep your expectations low about this first step in the appeals process. It's a necessary exercise, but not one that will always bring you satisfaction. While you are waiting to hear back from the HMO, assume that your appeal will be denied. Use the time that you are waiting to prepare for another round. The next best thing to do is write directly to the top doc in the organization—the medical director.

How Do I Write an Appeal Letter?

Make it your goal to write only one letter. The letter you write should have all the information the appeals board will need to decide on your case once and for all. With just one letter, you need to explain your condition, help them find a new perspective, and make them see you as a person. You will want to take time with your letter, and be sure to get some assistance.

Your letter to the medical director will be reviewed, along with your chart, by the director himself, UR doctors, and a utilization management committee. This committee may consist of independent doctors as well as the organization's own doctors. Dr. Feinberg serves on committees like these, and gets paid a small honorarium to give an independent opinion. These are good jobs for a doctor to get if the case is interesting, and most cases that make it to this level are very interesting.

We hear many concerns about these committees, about how they are structured in the HMO's favor. Texas was the first state to build a check against conflict of interest in the appeals process by requiring HMOs to allow review by an independent appeals board. Since this legislation passed, about 50 percent of the cases that get to that level are overturned. In the other half of these cases, the independent board agrees with the HMO. The split is pretty even—HMOs aren't doing a *great* job of providing medically necessary care, but they aren't exactly the monsters some reporters would have us believe.

By 2000, the National Association of Quality Assurance (NCQA) will accredit only those HMOs that allow independent review of cases under appeal. This means the NCQA will have to create a set of standards for reviewing organizations. Like we said earlier, the search for quality is making the appeals process ever more complicated, and there's no guarantee that a board is truly independent. The doctors involved all know each other. Some have business agreements on the side that may be perfectly legal, but which may dispose them to agree with the organization's original opinion. So even if you are sure that your appeal is going to an independent board, you still need to present the strongest case possible.

While making your strong case, you will also have to be brief.

Nothing will prejudice a committee against you like a long, rambling letter full of complaints and grievances. You should get right to the point, maintain a professional tone, and then ask for specific help. The best way to do this is to use the method you have already learned: HEAD.

Be sure to put a subject heading on your letter. "Re: Appeal for asthma treatment," or something similarly short and direct. On the next line, put your member ID number. Address the letter directly to a person—don't just write "Dear Medical Director" and leave it at that. You can get the medical director's name through the plan's toll-free hotline.

Start your letter with your identifying information from HEAD: "I am a fifty-five-year-old black female, employed by Millennia Cablevision as vice president of advertising, recently diagnosed with osteoarthritis in my left knee," for example. Earlier, we advised you to be frank about your sexual orientation with your doctor. Here, you don't have to do that unless you know that your illness is related to sexual activity. You can also probably skip the next stages of HEAD. The source of referral and the source of the history may not apply. Go directly to your chief complaint.

Now that you are in an appeal, your chief complaint is different from what you told your doctor. Tell the director why you are writing: "I am writing to appeal the denial of my treatment, an arthroscopy of the affected joint." Now state why you should get the treatment: "I am appealing on the grounds that this procedure is medically necessary, and that omission of this procedure will make my condition worse."

By the time the medical director has read this, you will have his full attention. You have used the exact language HMOs use to deny treatment. You have directly called their interpretation of your contract into question. You have presented yourself as someone who knows how to play the game. He will have to take you seriously.

Always avoid using phrases like "I think," "I believe," or "I request." If your doctor thinks, believes, or requests that you should get the treatment, you should say so, but the committee doesn't really care what *you* think. They deal in medical facts and opinions, not patients' intuitions.

A SAMPLE APPEAL LETTER

Dr. Donald Director
The Virtuous Medical Group
1000 Careaway Lane
Curetown, PA 01000

RE: Appeal for denied [condition and treatment]
      Member ID#: 888–888–888

Dear Dr. [Name of director]:

I am a [age, sex, race, employer, position]. I was diagnosed with [exact medical name of illness and exact location] on [date] by [name of HMO physician]. I am writing to appeal the denial of [exact name of treatment], denied to me on [date of denial].

I am appealing on the grounds that this procedure is medically necessary, and that the omission of this procedure will make [or has made] my condition worse.

My present illness started on [date] and has worsened to the point where [describe how it has gotten worse]. I have tried [If you have tried certain treatments and failed, detail these here. If you are still on a treatment, detail this here], but my condition has not been affected. My doctor recommended [name of denied treatment], but to my disappointment, this recommendation was denied by the Virtuous Medical Group on [date].

My present illness has had a serious effect on my quality of life. [Give examples of how the illness affects you, especially if it affects your work.]

The denied treatment was recommended by my doctor, and has also been recommended by [if you have a second opinion, mention this here. If you have treatment guidelines from the HMO or other medical organizations, mention these here.] Clearly, prevailing medical opinion sees the denied treatment as beneficial and necessary.

The denied treatment is also a covered benefit. The enclosed copy of my explanation of benefits [and/or Virtuous Medical Group's own guidelines] state that [quote from guidelines].

In summary, [denied treatment] should be allowed as soon as possible to prevent my condition from becoming worse. It is medically necessary and a covered benefit. I look forward to hearing from you by [allow a week to ten days, unless your condition is of a more serious or emergent nature].

A copy of this letter has been forwarded to [name and title of benefits manager or CFO], who handles employee benefits for my employer, [company name]. Thank you for your consideration.

Sincerely,

[Your name]

A SAMPLE APPEAL LETTER (continued)

Enclosures:

Medical report

Written opinion of Dr. [name of doctor]

[Name of organization]'s guidelines for treatment of [illness]

Page [page number] of Virtuous Medical Group's Explanation of Benefits

Copy of complete medical records

Cc: [name, title, and company name of employee benefits manager or CFO]

Now move on to the next stage of HEAD—history of present illness. Be sure to be very brief as you cover this. You want to get across how your condition has gotten worse without treatment. If you received some treatment, but were cut off, explain how this treatment benefited you and how you have gotten worse since the treatment stopped. That will explain why you feel it should continue. Provide the key dates: the first time you noticed symptoms, the first visit to your doctor for the problem, and the date of the denial.

Next, bring it all back to you by summarizing your current health as it relates to your problem. Give one or two examples of how this illness has affected your life: "I am currently unable to perform my job and support my children as a result of this condition," or "I am presently unable to perform daily tasks—shopping, cooking, cleaning—on my own." If, and only if, your condition is extremely serious, say "I understand that if this condition gets worse, I may die."

By covering your current health in this way, you have accomplished a lot. You have gotten the review committee members to see you as a person, you have explained how their decision will directly affect your life, and you have created sympathy. You have also given them a taste of what a jury might hear if the case ever gets that far. Examples like those above can be used to award damages. If you can create fear and sympathy in your medical director's heart at the same time, your appeal is virtually won.

Next, show support from other professionals. If you have the support of the HMO doctor who recommended the treatment, say that you do, and be sure to get documentation of his support. You can really get the committee's attention if you explain how the denial has inter-fered with your doctor-patient relationship. Lawsuits have been won on this basis.

If you have sought help from a nonnetwork doctor, and he agrees with your assessment, say so. Enclose his letter. If you have guidelines from non-HMO sources, say that you do, and enclose the guidelines with the relevant sections highlighted. Be sure to say where they come from.

Now show that you know your contract. You should have the HMO's denial form. You should also have your HMO's explanation of benefits or a summary description thereof. Compare the two by listing the reasons for denial, followed by the HMO's explanation of your ben-efit. If you have been denied something that your explanation of ben-efits says you should get, state that the denial contradicts the benefit. Describe how.

Summarize your case. Be sure to raise the question of medical necessity and assert strongly that what you seek is a covered benefit. Repeat the treatment or compensation you are seeking. Finally, ask for a response by a specific date. Allow one week if your condition is not life-threatening.

The last line of your letter will help your HMO put it all in perspec-tive. Let the plan administrators know that you are ready to get your employer involved. A simple sentence should do: "Please be informed that a copy of this letter has been sent to my employee benefits man-ager." Before you send the appeals letter, find out who the best contact person is at your company. It could be your human resources manager, your employee benefits manager, or even your CFO. Try to find out who selected your health plan, get his or her name, and be sure to men-tion it in your appeals letter. Be sure that your benefits manager gets updates about your appeal.

By taking this simple step, you hit the HMO where it really counts. In most cases, you are not the HMO's real consumer. Your employer is. Your employer has a contract with your health plan, and if that con-tract is terminated, your HMO takes a serious blow. If you let your HMO know that your employer is watching this appeal, even a treat-ment that costs thousands of dollars will begin to look like a bargain.

You will want to provide several documents with your letter. Enclose a copy of the denial, often called a "medial report." Provide a copy of any letters written on your behalf by advocates. These can be nonplan doctors, your own HMO doctor, or patient advocacy groups. Include copies of the HMO's own guidelines if you are sure that your denied treatment is covered by them. Include a copy of the relevant page from your explanation of benefits. Finally, and this should be at the bottom of your stack, include a copy of your medical records.

Yes, your HMO already has these. But the medical director will need to see your chart before he makes a decision. If you don't include your medical records, he will have to send off a request for the file to be transferred to his office. By the time it gets there, he will have forgotten

---

THE LEGAL OPTION

Suing your HMO can be an expensive, time-consuming option. It's best to hold this out as a last resort. Often there is a question of whether HMOs can be sued by patients at all. A lot of the confusion stems from interpretations of the Employee Retirement Income Security Act (ERISA), which simplified employee benefits regulations by removing them from state laws. In many cases, the employer's contract with the HMO allows only settlement by arbitration. As health care reform moves ahead on the state and federal level, it will probably become easier for patients to sue their HMOs, but we still feel that it's best to use the legal option only if all else has failed. Here are some tips for applying legal pressure to your health plan:

- Figure out what your case is worth in dollars. Before a lawyer will take a case, she has to be sure that it's worth her time and effort. Find out how much the treatment will cost if you get it on your own. Calculate missed work days and other real losses.

- Select a lawyer with relevant experience. Lawyers who specialize in personal injury, employment law, or malpractice suits will be best able to navigate the changing landscape of managed care.

- Don't be swayed by promises of large settlements. Many cases have ended with the patient compensated only for out-of-pocket health expenses. Many state regulations prohibit large punitive damages against managed care organizations. You could be left with legal bills just as large, or larger, than the cost of the treatment.

- Try to incorporate your lawyer into your appeal first. Sometimes a forceful letter from a good lawyer will be enough to bring your HMO around.

- Keep your employer up-to-date on your legal action. In some cases, employers can be held responsible for a health plan's actions. The court might see the health plan as an agent of the employer. This will motivate your employer to apply pressure of its own.

what the case was all about. It's much better if he can look at your medical records right away. He may come to a decision in your favor right there and then. He'll know he's dealing with a savvy, intelligent person, someone unlikely to be submitting an unreasonable request.

Your case is unique, but if you follow these general guidelines, you will make a powerful statement: You know your rights, you know your contract, and you know your condition. You won't lie down quietly and let the HMO line its pockets while your health deteriorates. You also show the HMO that you are cooperative, informed, and concerned. You aren't just looking to win. You simply want the best care.

WHERE CAN I GET HELP?

You are not alone in your appeal. As managed care covers more lives, state agencies, nonprofit organizations, and businesses are reaching out to patients in trouble. Your own research will uncover organizations that will give you advice and advocacy specific to your illness. Here are a few places to start:

The People's Medical Society
462 Walnut Street
Allentown, PA 18102
(610) 770–1670
www.peoplesmed.org

A widely respected nonprofit medical consumer advocacy group, established in 1983.

Families USA
1334 G Street NW
Washington, DC 20005
(202) 628–3030
www.familiesUSA.org

A consumer protection group. Supports patient's bill of rights and performs studies on managed care.

Patients Always First
7641 E. Gray Road, Suite G
Scottsdale, AZ 85260
(602) 493–9777
www.primenet.com/~paf

Provides consultation services for an annual subscription fee.

American Medical Consumers, Inc.
5415 Briggs Avenue
La Crescenta, CA 91214
(818) 957–3508
www.medconsumer.com

Offers organizational products and consultations for a fee.

CareCounsel, LLC
68 Mitchell Blvd., Suite 200
San Rafael, CA 94903
(415) 472–2366
www.carecounsel.com

Provides quality review of cancer cases for subscribers.

American Health Decisions
See website for an affiliate in your area
www.ahd.org

A nonprofit coalition that provides information on current issues in managed care.

When Should I Leave My Health Plan?

At the very end of the appeals line is the possibility of switching plans. For most of us, it's a very remote possibility. Since most patients get their insurance through their employer, they can, at most, chose between two or three plans. Many employers offer only one plan. This is why the health care industry hasn't fully embraced the quality issue. They know that most patients are stuck.

You should make every effort to work with what you have. If you can turn your doctor into your ally, use HEAD to make sure nothing is missed, stay on top of your preventive plan, and do your research, you should be able to make even the worst HMO work for you. But you may reach a point where you realize that the quality of care you are receiving, even after all your best efforts, isn't worth the money you or your employer pays. If you have the option, you may choose to shop for a new plan.

Watch for these warning signs. If you notice these problems, it may be time to switch.

- The HMO repeatedly loses paperwork. The information in your file directs your care. It can save your life. If your HMO constantly misplaces your file, or if you find paperwork missing from your file, this should tell you something. Your HMO doesn't have the organizational skills to provide good care. Don't wait for a medical problem to arise. Start looking elsewhere.

- You've tried several incompetent doctors. If Dr. X was a drunk, Dr. Y was rude, and Dr. Z was incompetent, your HMO may have a problem attracting and keeping the best doctors. Take a look around.

- You don't get consistent care. An HMO may start out with the best intentions. But if it starts to lose money, gets caught up in a merger, or begins downsizing, you may notice a change in quality. Find out what's going on. If it's not going to get better, start packing.

- You get repeated denials for even minor procedures. One of the most unethical practices of managed care is to deny all expensive treatments, and then allow denials to be overturned in appeal. The HMO violates its own rules in the hopes that a large number of patients will just accept denials of treatment. If you have to appeal everything you need, it's time to hit the road.

- You get overreaching denials. You should be able to understand why you were denied. Remember, medical necessity can be seen many different ways. But if it looks like the reasons for denial were forced, if someone had to really make an effort to come up with reasons to deny you care, there may be a serious problem with the way the plan is run. If it happens more than once, check out your other options.

- Your life is threatened. Bottom line: your life is more important than your money. If you just can't get proper treatment with your HMO, find a way to switch to a more comprehensive plan, even if it's more expensive.

I Give Up! How Do I Choose a New Health Plan?

If you are in a position to choose, and most of us aren't, you will be barraged with promises and statistics. Most of this information, unfortunately, has little to do with you. There really isn't a simple way for consumers to evaluate a health plan. In the end, you will have to pay more attention to your own needs than to the information in an HMO's marketing campaign or the fact that it may be independently accredited.

The National Committee for Quality Assurance (NCQA) has taken the lead in evaluating and accrediting health plans. But the NCQA has its critics. The accreditation is completely voluntary. Only a plan that thinks it can live up to the NCQA's standards will attempt to get accreditation. The NCQA gets a large portion of its operating budget from accreditation fees, opening it up to charges of conflicts of interest. And the board of the NCQA is largely composed of health industry insiders. Still, it is for now the biggest and best game in town.

Employers find NCQA data useful, as do reporters and consumer review studies. But it is of limited use to the consumer. Many of the benchmarks reported by the NCQA can offer insight into how well a population is being treated, but they don't say how *you* will be treated. For example, childhood immunization rates reported by the NCQA can tell a health plan administrator how well his plan is doing in the preventive treatment arena. They might make you confident that a plan cares about its population. But no HMO will refuse to immunize your child if you demand it.

Most of the NCQA benchmarks are based on noncontroversial guidelines for treatment. They don't address specific problems, and they won't address your concerns. If you are choosing a health plan, take a look at the NCQA data for your plan. You can find it on the World Wide Web at www.ncqa.org. But try to look past that data to your own needs.

What's Most Important to Me?

This is the key question to answer when choosing a health plan. What do you need from a health plan? Just a yearly checkup? An extensive treatment for chronic illness? What are you willing to pay? How important is customer service to you? Are you willing to put up with a bit of bureaucracy to pay a bit less? How important is it for you to see just one doctor? If you live in New York and work in New Jersey, can you see doctors in either state? Take all of your needs into account. An HMO will be a part of your life—investigate all the ways it can affect you.

You can evaluate your medical needs using HEAD and the risk assessment plan given in appendix B. Take this to your prospective health plan and ask direct questions. Do they have a program in place to deal with your condition or your screening needs? See if you can get a copy of their treatment guidelines for that illness. Compare these to guidelines from other sources. How do the prospective plan's guidelines stack up? Where are they lacking? Are you willing to live without certain treatment?

If you have a chronic condition that needs a large medical team, think about the network structure of your prospective health plan. A loose network, like an IPA or PPO, might be great if you value choice. But a tight, integrated structure, like in a staff or group model HMO, might make it easier for you to build a team.

If you have a preexisting condition, find out if you will be barred from the plan or charged a higher rate. Don't try to hide your condition during your application. It's a very bad idea to lie about health matters to your HMO. It will usually come back to haunt you.

If you have a strong need for customer service, place phone calls to the prospective plan posing as a member. How are the operators? Are they organized? Do they answer your questions? Are they friendly?

Are you willing to put up with slow or cursory customer service in exchange for a low monthly payment or a network of great doctors? Managed care is a world of compromises. Unless you are willing to pay top dollar, you will find that getting attention in one area will mean sacrificing quality in another. There is no way around this, but you can find a plan that works for you if you are clear about what you need.

How Do I Research My Choices?

Once you have established what you need, it will be easy for you to research your choices. Data provided by the NCQA will make more sense. Your questions will become more focused. You are ready to find the answers.

They won't have professional assessments, but your friends and coworkers are a great source of information on a prospective health plan. Take someone who is on the plan you are considering to lunch. Ask her everything you can. If she is healthy, she probably will be perfectly happy with her plan, but try to go beyond her surface impressions. Why did she choose this plan? How are the doctors? How are the reception staff? Has she ever had any problems, even small ones? Think about whom you are talking to. Is she easy to please? Or is she a demanding consumer? How closely will your experience match hers?

Your employee benefits manager can also be a great source of information on a plan. He will have heard marketing and sales pitches from all the plans, but he also will have heard employee complaints. Is the plan living up to its promises? Where has it fallen short? Which plan did he choose for himself? Why?

There are benefits and pitfalls in choosing a plan based on a single doctor. Having a good relationship with your doctor will open the doors to a good relationship with your HMO, so you might find a winning plan just by finding a good doctor. On the other hand, your doctor may leave the HMO or be delisted at any time, leaving you back where you started. If you get a list of doctors from a prospective plan, don't make a decision based on that list alone.

Call the doctor you have in mind. Make sure she is still on that plan and is accepting new patients from it. You might even get information from your doctor's support staff. What do they think of the HMO? Does the plan pay its bills on time? Does it deny many referrals? Unlike the doctor, members of her support staff usually aren't under contracts that prevent them from discussing the plan frankly.

As you ask these questions, don't expect an interview with your prospective doctor. She doesn't have time to sit down with you and discuss the individual merits of your prospective plan. She won't appreciate an approach that makes you appear distrustful. She's trained in treating patients, not in selling herself to patients.

Take a look at what's happening to your prospective HMO in the business world. If it has experienced a recent merger, its organization may be in disarray. If it's in the process of downsizing, be very wary of overworked doctors and administrators. If it is going through a period of aggressive growth, it may be making promises that it can't keep down the road. You want an HMO that is stable, and has been stable for some time.

Again, pay attention to your medical needs. Pepper your prospective HMO with phone calls about its treatment plans for your condition. Since health plan benefits are so complicated, you may get different answers each time you call. If this happens, ask to speak to the person in charge. Give them some time to get back to you with a *definitive* answer.

Finally, always take the HMO's own marketing literature with a grain of salt. It's never going to be as good as it sounds. You can look at the explanation of benefits booklet, or the new member summary, but there's always a much bigger set of rules tucked away at corporate headquarters that you may never be able to see. When you look at the HMO's promises, turn them into specific questions about your condition or potential condition. Always bring it back to your needs.

We believe that health plans will become more generic as accreditation becomes more commonplace, as health care becomes more regulated, and as consumers demand better care. We are approaching a standard that plans will have to live up to if they want to stay in business. When this happens, the only difference between one HMO and another will be convenience.

We also believe that you can get a high standard of care, even now, from just about any health plan. If you use HEAD, build a relationship with your doctor, prevent illness, and do your research when you do get sick, you can get the maximum of care from even the stingiest HMO. Being alert to your own condition and needs is far better than shopping around for a new plan. Refusing to take no for an answer from your current plan is far better than switching to another plan that may tell you the same thing.

What Have I Accomplished?

When you get through to your HMO with an intelligent appeal, you have done much more than win. You have set your standards and defined your boundaries. You have continued your research into your condition by establishing what is and isn't medically necessary. It gets better. When you complete a successful appeal, you will have gotten individualized care from a large organization driven by statistics. That can be a powerfully good feeling.

But when you appeal a decision by your health plan, or when you finally give up and take your money elsewhere, you are doing more than getting the best care for yourself. The question of what HMOs are supposed to do is still open. The term "medical necessity" is still undefined. When you push the issue of quality, you are contributing, in a small way, to a national debate over what quality in health care means. You have joined a chorus of concerned patients who refuse to be pushed aside by profit-driven health care.

In the next chapters, we will discuss the special needs of children, seniors, and psychiatric patients in HMOs. These are the groups that need the most individualized care, and so they are most often the groups that get neglected. If you don't fall into any of these groups, take a look at these chapters anyway. You may someday have to be an advocate for someone else.

~ 8 ~

Managed Child Care
Guiding Your Child through Your HMO

QUESTIONS THIS CHAPTER ANSWERS

◆ How will my HMO treat my child?

◆ How do I prepare for my child's appointment?

◆ What records should I keep?

◆ When should I take my child to the ER?

◆ How do I use HEAD with my child's doctor?

◆ How do doctors assess and decide on treatment for children?

Of all the lives a managed care organization covers, none are more precious than those of the children. If you believe HMO advertising, you would think that they fully agree. Children are featured prominently in managed care ad campaigns—we see a cute child smiling at a friendly doctor who smiles back as he places a gentle hand on the kid's shoulder. Ads like these get us right in the heart, even if we aren't parents. It's easy to see why.

The reality, of course, can be very different. HMOs are great at caring for healthy adults, but children far too often fall through the cracks. Of all the HMO horror stories we have heard, the most compelling always involve children. One of those stories was told to us by a woman we will call Dora.

Dora moved into a new house shortly after her child, "Jasper," was born. The house was a bargain, but old, and in desperate need of renovation. Knowing that lead paint, which is often found in older homes, tastes sweet to children, Dora wouldn't sign the papers until she had the seller's assurance that the paint falling off the walls was safe. The seller told her it was, and she moved in.

It wasn't long after Jasper started to crawl that she noticed he was sleeping more than normal. She asked her HMO doctor about it during a regular "well baby" exam, and expressed her concern about the paint. The doctor noted that Jasper's weight and growth were normal. He was eating regularly. Taking a lead level test would involve expensive blood work. Everything else seemed fine, so Jasper's doctor decided against the test. "Come back in a year," he told her, "and if he still has low energy, we'll do the test."

Jasper continued to grow normally and eat regularly, but Dora knew something was wrong. His daycare teachers reported that he didn't participate in activities. He preferred to sleep or sit quietly. He had a burst of energy in the afternoon when Dora picked him up, but within an hour, he was again listless and lethargic. "His arms had no strength in them," Dora told us. "They felt like wet noodles."

Nine months later, Dora couldn't take it anymore. She went back to the doctor, and told him that if he still couldn't recommend the test, she would pay for it herself. As if finally sensing her urgency, the doctor asked for the test. When the blood work came back, he saw that Jasper's lead level was off the chart.

The doctor considered hospitalization, and then a treatment called chelation. The HMO's information resources kicked into gear, and Dora found out from a nurse that she could order a free test from the government to check her paint. The health plan was now ready to help, but Dora still feels that all this could have been averted if the test had been provided when she first expressed her concern.

Jasper is fine. His lead levels miraculously and inexplicably dropped before he had to undergo any invasive procedures. As he develops, he shows no signs of damage. Dora, however, has to live with this memory. She's angry with the doctor, as she should be, but says that the guilt is an even heavier burden: "I wish I had followed my intuition. Unfortunately, because I didn't act on it, I exposed him to nine more months of lead poisoning."

As doctors, we can see the mistakes Dora's HMO doctor made. Sleep patterns are an important part of any child's medical history, which we will discuss later in this chapter. This doctor didn't ask the right questions. But in the time-compressed era of managed care, you can't always count on doctors to ask the right questions. In some plans, you might not even get to see a pediatrician right away. When something is wrong with your child, you can't afford to get the brush-off. You have to make sure that you give the doctor all the information he needs right from the beginning.

"I wish that doctors would listen to mothers," Dora told us. "They know their kids. They know when something is wrong." She's absolutely right. You know when something is wrong. The trick is to get your HMO to pay attention. In this chapter, we will show you how.

How Will My HMO Treat My Child?

An HMO can give your child a great start. Almost all of a pediatrician's work is devoted to "well baby" checkups, which fits right in with the idea of health maintenance. Catching problems before they become damaging and expensive saves your child from suffering, and saves the HMO money.

Just think: under fee-for-service, there was no financial incentive to make sure a child got immunizations. It only happened for social and humanitarian reasons. Hospitals would actually make more money if a child got sick from an easily preventable disease. Now, under managed care, the opposite is true. Furthermore, the NCQA and consumer protection groups grade HMOs on how many of their covered kids are immunized. And of course, doctors and nurses feel good about themselves when they immunize children. A high immunization rate can boost morale throughout the organization.

In thinking about your child's care, think in terms of prevention first. Always try to get your HMO to adopt the same attitude. In the best HMOs this won't be difficult—they are learning how to do this on their own. Harvard-Pilgrim Health Care in Boston, widely considered one of the best, achieved stunning results in treating childhood asthma by training patients and their parents in the use of peak-flow meters and inhalers. Even young children can take control of their own health with this simple device that tells them when to expect an attack, and how severe it will be. Harvard Pilgrim's inpatient admissions for childhood asthma dropped by 86 percent, while ER visits dropped by 79 percent after the program was instituted. The health plan is saving money, and the kids it covers are staying out of the hospital. In most cases, everybody wins when prevention is given top priority.

Managed care is also less likely to push for unnecessary interventions and procedures. In the past, children have been the recipients of all sorts of questionable care. Remember how doctors removed the tonsils of almost an entire generation? Looking back, it seems almost insane, a medical fad that came and went. We now know that tonsils are an important part of the immune system, and their removal should not be taken lightly.

Since parents are so concerned about their children's health, they have been willing to go along with just about anything that doctors recommend. The tympasoctomy is another example. Millions of children have had a tube inserted into their ears to allow problem fluids to drain out, even when there was no concrete proof that this procedure helped. Fee-for-service doctors, however, were slow to respond to these findings.

Another example: We live in the only country in the world that routinely performs circumcisions for nonreligious reasons. It's the number-one inpatient procedure in the country. But it's one that's frequently questioned. In 1999, the Pediatric Society, after years of consideration and investigation, finally came out against the procedure. For better or worse, this will force a change. HMOs just won't cover circumcisions if an independent group like the Pediatric Society is against it. After all, each procedure can cost over $1,500 in an inpatient setting.

We believe there are still questions to be answered about circumcision. In some cases a tympasoctomy is beneficial. Sometimes a tonsillectomy is necessary. But at least someone is questioning these procedures. To be honest, doctors in the past weren't doing a great job of questioning procedures on their own, especially when it came to kids. Now managed care is forcing all of us to think before we let a doctor cut.

That's the good news about letting managed care cover your child. Now for the downside. While HMOs can be great at preventing illness and weeding out unnecessary procedures for kids, they can be horrible at treating sick children. Kids get sicker more quickly than adults. If the problem isn't caught and treated right the first time, a child's normal development can be sidetracked. The necessary rapid response doesn't quite fit with the way HMOs normally do business.

A sick kid doesn't have time for paperwork delays. You can't waste time attempting to treat a sick kid with an inexpensive treatment and come back to the more expensive treatment if it doesn't work. You can't wait on getting the right test. There's a larger margin of error in adults. They can survive a minor mistake without suffering long-term effects. But you can't cut corners when you are treating a sick child.

Managed care organizations also aren't their best when dealing with rare diseases or specialized treatments, even in adults. With kids, they are worse. A pediatrician is a specialist, just like a pulmonologist (lung specialist). A pulmonologist who further specializes in treating children is a *subspecialist*. There aren't that many out there, and their fees are high. It's very unlikely that your HMO will have a pediatric pulmonologist in its network. They might try to send children to an in-network adult pulmonologist who has little experience with pediatric cases. This is usually a bad choice.

Finally, and this is where you have to be at your best, many child patients can't talk to doctors. Children who can talk haven't lived in their bodies long enough to really know when something is wrong. They don't have the same communication tools as adults. That creates a problem for managed care. In chapter 3, when you were learning how to use HEAD, we explained how a health plan can save money by getting information from a history rather than from a test. It's a good idea. Patients avoid invasive procedures, and HMOs save money. But the same mode of operation just won't work with children.

Children depend on you for food, warmth, and love. In managed care, they also depend on you to explain to the doctor what is wrong. If the doctor misses an important part of the history or fails to ask an important question, like Dora's doctor did, the child depends on you to fill in the blanks. In fee-for-service, Dora's simple complaint of her child's listlessness would have led to a battery of tests. In managed care, parents like Dora have to give more detailed information. Through the child's history, which the parent provides, you have to demonstrate that the test is medically necessary.

You have already learned HEAD, and you can use it for your child as well as yourself. But when giving your child's history, you will need to address specific concerns. The most important things to cover in a pediatric history are sleep, growth, eating and digestion, crying, patterns of irritability, and developmental milestones. Just as you would for yourself, the best time to start thinking about these issues and gathering the necessary information is before you go to the doctor's office.

How Do I Prepare for My Child's Appointment?

Your child may be too young to speak, or she may be too young to fully express her symptoms, but you can take clues from her activities and behavior. The doctor will need this information to make a good decision. The more organized you are, the better you will be at convincing the doctor that there is a problem.

What if Dora had been able to explain in greater detail how weak her child had become? Instead of saying, "Jasper seems to be sleeping more than normal," she might have said, "Jasper has been sleeping an average of twenty hours a day, where he used to sleep sixteen hours a day. He only maintains about one hour of activity a day, and no more than fifteen minutes at a time." There's no way that a doctor, upon hearing this, would doubt that something is wrong. There's no way to write you off as an anxious parent. But the only way you can protect your child with this information is to keep records and prepare for the visit.

What Records Should I Keep?

Parents naturally keep some records of their child's development. Notches cut into a door frame to measure height, photo albums of special events, or videotape of a baby's first steps are just a few examples of the records that keep our memories fresh and allow us to share our excitement with others. It's an important part of being a parent.

The records you keep for your visit shouldn't be so different. They are there to keep your memory fresh and enable you to communicate your concern with your child's doctor. They can even help you spot potential problems long before they become serious. Aside from the record keeping you should do when an illness becomes apparent, which we covered in chapter 3, you will want to pay special attention to the following patterns. Any good doctor will want to know about these, and it's a good idea to be prepared with an answer.

Sleep Patterns

Infants, as you probably know, seem to sleep almost all the time. That, in itself, is nothing to worry about. But even if you don't think there's a problem, it's still a good idea to keep track, even in a general way, of how much downtime your baby needs. If she's following a normal pattern, that's good for the doctor to know. He can rule out some problems just from this simple fact.

If you want to take this very seriously, write down your estimates for your baby's total hours of sleep per day. Also take note of how much sleep he takes at a time, and how long he stays awake between naps. As your child gets older, he will sleep less. If you don't notice a gradual lessening of naptime, or if you notice a sudden change in his patterns, take note, and let your doctor know.

If you find you have missed keeping complete records, don't worry. If you can provide a good record for the two weeks prior to the office visit, that's still a big help for your doctor. If you miss keeping a two-week record, think hard about your child's sleep patterns before the visit. Take some notes based on your memory. Try to be as accurate as you can. At minimum, when the doctor asks you "How often does he sleep?" you want to be able to say more than "Oh, he sleeps all the time."

Growth Patterns

Keeping track of growth patterns can be fun for both kids and parents, and they are also a part of your child's clinical picture. Your doctor will measure and weigh your child as well, so your records will be used to track the pattern between office visits. They will also alert you to changes that you may need to bring to your doctor's attention. If for example, your child is eating more than ever, but her weight is dropping, this could suggest a problem. If increased growth doesn't match increased sleep, this might tell your doctor something.

In the early months of life, you can see changes in weight and slight changes in height week by week. Later, you may want to take your measurements on a monthly or bimonthly basis. Keep track of the figures and dates in the same place you keep your notes on sleep patterns. Be sure to bring these records to the doctor with you.

Eating and Digestion

In the first few years of life, you should discuss your infant's diet at every visit. Be prepared to tell your doctor how often your child eats, how long he nurses or how much he takes from the bottle, and any problems with nursing or bottle feeding. All babies "spit up," and new parents are usually surprised at how often this happens. It's probably not a cause for concern, but your doctor can only be sure if you can give her an idea of how often this happens and to what extent.

If you are using formula, be sure to bring the package with you so the doctor can check the ingredients. Also bring any diet supplements—vitamins and iron supplements are particularly important. Remember, if you are nursing, your diet is your child's. Bring any prescription drugs, over-the-counter or herbal medicines, or vitamins that *you* are taking as well.

As your child is weaned, be sure to take note of these important dates. When did you start, how long did it take before your child accepted it, and how did you do it? After your child is on solid foods, you won't have to keep as close a record of his eating habits. But take note of what you see: What does he like or not like? Does he seem to eat too much or too little? Examine your own attitudes toward food as well.

If your child has a problem specifically related to eating and digestion, you may be asked to keep a seven- or fourteen-day "diet diary." If you notice a problem, don't wait until you are asked. If you can present this diary to the doctor at the same time you present him with the problem, you can save time—and maybe even avoid a second visit.

Crying Patterns

How does a parent know when a baby is in pain? Sometimes the only way to tell is if the baby is crying, but babies cry day and night. If your baby's crying is causing you concern and you want to relate this to your doctor, you may have to convince him that it goes beyond what is normal. If you notice your baby crying more than usual, start taking notes. How much has the crying increased? How much more frequently does it occur? Does it change in quality? Does it have a different pitch? Have the usual comforts stopped working?

You are taking notes to make sure a busy HMO doctor or nurse does not dismiss you. They hear complaints about babies crying day after day. Some babies are colicky, and will just cry. But some complaints may be tied to real problems that should be investigated. If you can present your case in a way that shows you have already thought about it, your doctor will have to look harder.

Developmental Milestones

Parents celebrate when a child takes her first steps, when her first teeth appear, or when she says her first word. Doctors watch for these milestones as well. Regular development indicates a normal, healthy child. A delayed milestone, however, may indicate a problem that requires further investigation.

It's your doctor's job to ask about and record these milestones. But you can help the process along, spare him guesswork, and save valuable time if you keep a record of those events that he will be sure to ask about. Take note of the following milestones. Write down when they occurred, and mention any problems or symptoms the child had at that time.

- How old was the child when teeth first appeared? How old when he lost his first "baby tooth"? What symptoms did he experience during teething?

- When did your child first hold up her head without help?

- How old was he when he sat up, all on his own, completely without support?

- How old was she when she first walked without help?

- How old was he when he said his first word?

These are records you should keep whether your child is sick or well. Understand that by keeping these records, you aren't just making your doctor's job easier. You are, and she will appreciate it, but that's not the point. The real reason for keeping track is for the benefit of your child. You are tracking her health. If you can do a thorough job, managed care will respond when you ask for help.

How Do I Prepare My Child for My Visit?

In an HMO, the best care goes to the patients best able to express themselves. That's why, in chapter 3, we showed you exactly how to present your case to the doctor. But we don't expect you to teach HEAD to your kid. You will have to serve as advocate for your child. The items in HEAD are just as important for children, but you will have to do much of the talking.

Before you go for your visit, ask your child some questions. Pretend you are the doctor, and try to anticipate, from what you have learned in chapter 3, what your doctor might ask. Get your child to talk to you about the problem. Then write down exactly what she says. When doctors take a medical history, they try to use the patient's exact words, but there's always a chance that younger patients will get nervous and clam up in the examining room. If this happens, you will be ready to give the doctor the description your child gave you when she was relaxed and looking for help.

Encourage your child to point to the pain or discomfort. Ask him what it feels like—is it burning? Pounding? Sharp? Use "kid words" and hand motions. Get him to compare it to other sensations that he has had in the past. Does it feel like the time you slipped on the kitchen floor? Or does it feel like the last tummy ache you had? Is it worse? Or is it not as bad?

Be sure to take note of what makes the condition worse or better. Keep asking your child if it gets better or worse when she does things like lie down, stand up, run, walk, or watch TV. Get your child thinking about what makes it better or worse. Keep track of these possible factors by writing them down.

Some kids will be able to answer all the questions we have given you in HEAD. Some will only be able to answer a few. You know your child best, and will be able to judge from his answers what you should ask next. The important thing at this stage is to prepare your child for the same questions when the doctor asks them.

You can also help prepare your child for the exam. A sick child can get very nervous in the hospital environment, especially when a stranger, who may be rushed, starts looking down his throat and poking his abdomen. Before you go to the exam, take some time to make your child feel at ease.

With your child's favorite doll or stuffed animal, show her what the doctor is going to do, what he is going to look at, and how it might feel. At each visit, the doctor will take a temperature, height and weight measurements, blood pressure, and heart rate. As you act out the exam with your child, a Popsicle stick can serve as a thermometer, and you can find a plastic stethoscope in just about any toy store. Taking blood pressure can be uncomfortable for children—you will want to explain what is going to happen. Show her how it will feel by lightly squeezing her arm. If she wants to try it on her doll, get her to tie a sock around her doll's arm. Get your child to play doctor on her own with the stuffed animal. By the time she's ready to go, the exam will be familiar and unthreatening.

Don't lie to your child about how injections and blood samples won't hurt. They do. Instead, emphasize how it will be over in just a second. You will be there, and you will make sure everything turns out all right. Explain how that little bit of pain from the needle will prevent worse pain down the road.

All this assumes that your child is old enough to talk. You will need a different strategy for infants. You want to be able to provide objective observations that point to subjective feelings—what your baby is experiencing. An example would be that your child, who used to smile all the time, hasn't smiled since the illness started. Or perhaps she hasn't cooed since the problem became apparent. Maybe picking her up, which used to comfort her, now makes her cry. Has the quality of her crying changed? This is important to note. Does it now sound more like a shriek? Or is it more like sobbing?

You can pick up all sorts of clues from changes in your child's behavior. These clues will allow your doctor to go quickly to a possible diagnosis. Being organized and ready with these clues is vital in a managed care environment. The last thing you want is the brush-off. If you aren't ready to present a complete picture to a rushed HMO doctor, that's exactly what you will get.

What Should I Take to My Child's Visit?

In addition to your notes and records—a description of the symptom in your child's own words and the history you have taken of your child's sleep, growth, eating, and crying patterns—there are a couple of items you should pack for your visit.

First and foremost, take your child's medications with you. We have mentioned this before, but it is very important. In a plastic bag, place all your child's prescription medications and any over-the-counter drugs or vitamins she takes. The doctor needs to be able to see the exact drug and the exact dose. There's always a chance you could forget a detail that's on the bottle, so instead of making a list or trying to memorize everything, just empty out your child's medicine cabinet. Nursing mothers should bring all of their medications, vitamins, and over-the-counter drugs. All of these can come through the mother's milk in a very pure form—and can possibly lead to drug interactions in the baby.

When you get to your doctor's office, there's a good chance you will have to wait. A waiting room can feel like a jail cell to a child. It's dull, there's nothing to do, and the chairs are uncomfortable. We know how frustrating it is for an adult to wait for a doctor who's a half-hour behind schedule. It's worse when you have a stir-crazy kid looking for stimulation in a bland environment.

Be prepared for a long wait. Bring toys and your child's favorite doll or stuffed animal. Use the time to explain again to your child what the doctor is going to do and how he's going to make your child feel better. When your child gets bored with this drill, he can entertain himself with the toys you've brought.

What Do I Say When I Call My HMO?

Most parents don't need to be encouraged to call their HMO when their child is sick. They don't need to be discouraged, either. Children's illnesses can quickly develop into serious problems. You should never be afraid to call your doctor or your HMO if you suspect something is wrong.

But you can't expect the best service over the phone. Doctors can do quite a bit with descriptions of symptoms, but it's all guesswork until they see the patient themselves. Besides, you may not be able to reach a doctor. If you call your HMO's urgent care center, you can't assume that the person who picks up the phone is trained to answer your questions.

You can assume that they are overworked. There's a chance they don't want to hear your concerns. In a study conducted by the University of Pittsburgh, researchers posing as parents of a five-week-old child with clear warning signs of meningitis called sixty-one hospitals; only thirty-two hospitals insisted that they bring the child in immediately. That scares us.

It's a common story: a worried parent calls the emergency room and describes a child's symptoms, only to be told not to worry. The

---

MEDICAL ALERTS FOR CHILDREN

Fever
Any fever in a child under a month old is serious. A newborn infant's blood/brain barrier is not fully developed, and any infection can lead to severe problems. There may be nothing to worry about, but a doctor's attention, and quite possibly lab work, is needed.

Dehydration
Just like adults suffering from a "common cold," children need to keep their fluid levels up. However, in children, dehydration can happen very quickly and with fewer warning signs. Keep track of how many times you are changing your baby's diapers. If the diapers are dry and you aren't changing them as much as you used to, he might be dehydrated. If the amount of vomit is close to the volume of feedings, watch the situation carefully. Check for skin elasticity. If you pinch your child lightly, does the skin snap back as it did when he was healthy?

---

problem doesn't go away, and the parent calls again, only to receive a similar answer. Finally, when the parent can't take it anymore, she brings the child in and a doctor says, "This is serious. Why didn't you bring him in sooner?" The parent looks around the room. Someone else in here is going to need medical attention.

A parent who told us one of these stories summed it up perfectly: "I kept calling, and I kept getting the feeling that I was asking permission." You are not asking permission. If it's clear to you, as a "prudent layperson," that your child needs immediate medical attention, you shouldn't need permission. The purpose of your call is to gather information to help you make the right decision. Don't let the person on the other end of the line make that decision for you.

Here are some things to keep in mind when making that call:

- Let the person you are speaking with know that you are concerned, but not panicked. People who have seen lots of overreacting parents tend to think that they all overreact.

- Find out who you are talking to. Make sure you at least have a nurse on the line. See if you can get a pediatric nurse.

- Use HEAD. Give your child's identifying information, chief complaint, and history of the present illness.

- If the HMO representative taking your call does not recommend bringing your child in, get more information. Don't hang up until you have some answers and a plan: What do you think it is? What else could it be? How can this be treated at home?

- Be sure to ask what to watch out for. Are there any other symptoms that should be taken as warning signs? What's the normal course of this illness? When should my child be over it?

When you hang up the phone, don't accept what the HMO recommends without thinking about it yourself. You called to get information. Now make sure that information is appropriate to the sick child in front of you. There are certain symptoms that would be no concern for an adult, but deserve a doctor's attention in infants, no matter what you might have been told. If these conditions are all there, you have told the whole story, and you are still being told not to bring the child in, talk to the person in charge. Bring the child in anyway. You may have to appeal it later, but your peace of mind and your child's health are worth the trouble.

How Do I Use HEAD with My Child's Doctor?

When a doctor takes a child's medical history, she follows the same form, asks many of the same questions, and is looking for the same clues. There are special needs that have to be addressed, but the basic form and idea are the same. If you can do it for yourself, you can do it for your kid.

But the biggest difference to the doctor, if the child is old enough to talk, is that he is getting information from two sources. This means that in the space of a ten-minute visit, he has to hear both your version of the illness and the child's. That means it's more important than ever to keep the visit organized—not for your doctor's sake, but for the sake of your child.

Using HEAD will get your child the best medical service managed care can deliver, but it also does something else. Your concerns will be taken seriously. Too many doctors are predisposed to take worried parents less seriously than they should. They walk into a situation assuming the child they are about to see suffers from only a minor complaint that has been blown out of proportion by the parent. This kind of inclination should never affect a medical decision, but like all prejudices, it's hard to get past.

When you use HEAD, you can sail past this obstacle easily. Sure you are concerned, but you also come equipped with a complete history that proves you need medical answers. It shows that you are acting on information you have gathered, and not just out of fear. By the time you get to the decision, there will be a team—you, your doctor, and in some cases even your child.

Identifying Information: Who's the Kid?

This should come from the parent. Just as in the adult history, you should give the child's age, race, gender, place of birth, and the parent's religion. You should add to this information the following:

- Nickname (helps the doctor talk to the child).
- Parents' marital status (lets the doctor know what questions to ask in taking the family history).
- Parents' names (helps the doctor tie your records to your child's).
- Adoption. If the child was adopted, it's vital that the doctor has this information. Medical records from the adoption agency are essential.
- Parents' occupation (helps the doctor establish or rule out possible environmental factors).

Here again, don't let the personal nature of this information get in the way of medicine. Being up-front about your religion, for example, will help both you and your doctor avoid uncomfortable situations later. There can also be significant medical clues contained in information like your child's ethnic background. It's not a political, religious, or racial issue when you are in the examining room. It's about your child's health and well-being.

Chief Complaint: Why Are You Here?

Whenever possible, this should first come from the child. Good doctors make every effort to put down the chief complaint in the patient's own words. This allows them to move from the subjective—what the child feels—to the objective, or what the outward signs are.

If your child can express his own chief complaint, let him go first. Then take your turn.

If your child did a good job with the chief complaint, all you need to add is why you decided to come in now. What did you notice that meant you couldn't wait? If your child didn't express herself as well as you know she can, let her try again. Perhaps she told you something earlier that she isn't telling the doctor now. You can ask her to repeat what she told you to the doctor. This allows her to explain the complaint in her own words, and also lets her know that she can tell the doctor anything that she tells you. This all contributes to building trust.

If a third party—a teacher, babysitter, or relative—first noticed the problem, be sure to say so. It's always important for the doctor to know where the information came from. The third party may be able to complete the picture the doctor is drawing in her mind. The source of the information can be as important as the information itself.

Present Illness: Where, When, Why, and How Does It Hurt?

This information should come from the child whenever possible, and should be added to by the parent. Review the present illness section in chapter 3. There is a specific way doctors describe symptoms that works as well for children as it does for adults. The eight parts of a symptom, as we detailed in chapter 3, are as follows:

- Location
- Quality
- Quantity or severity
- Timing
- Setting
- Factors
- Associated symptoms

It can be tough to get this information out of a kid. That's why we recommended earlier in this chapter that you talk with your child before the visit. The doctor is responsible for asking the right questions, but the inescapable truth of managed care is that patients have to be ready with accurate and informative answers. None of the above parts of a symptom can be skipped. Each part will help lead the doctor quickly to an exact diagnosis.

There is one piece of information to add to the history of the present illness: *Response of family members to the illness*. When we described how to talk about quantity or severity with your doctor, we recommended that you detail the effect on your life. For example, in describing your own illness you might say, "The problem has gotten so bad that I've had to take time off work." For your child, the doctor should hear about how the problem has affected the child's activities, but he should also hear about how it has affected other family members. For example, "Junior told me that he can't take part in physical education at school. I've been worried sick about him. My wife has been late for work three times this last week because he needs our help and comfort three to four times a night. Our other son, who is six, has been depressed and distant ever since this started."

The doctor can take clues from this description of how the illness affects other family members. The figure "three to four times a night" is a measurement of the severity of the problem. The fact that the sibling is depressed may point to a developing psychological condition that requires intervention, or a physical problem—maybe he's getting sick as well. A sick child affects an entire family. Knowing exactly in what way can help the doctor determine the cause of the problem.

Even if there are no clues in your description of the family response, it still helps. It allows the doctor to see you as people in need. It motivates him to get to a cure. It brings out sympathy and compassion. It will help win the doctor over to your side, where he will fight against cost-cutting to get your child the very best care. Response of family members is always relevant.

Past Health: What's Happened Before?

This should come from the parent. A child's past health history is slightly different from an adult's. While both adults and children may be asked about accidents, hospitalizations, and psychiatric conditions, doctors need details on the early stages of a child's life. It wasn't that long ago, medically speaking, and there may be some unresolved issues that now show up as illness.

Birth History

If your child is two years old or younger, make sure you are prepared to tell your doctor about the following elements of the child's birth history:

- Prenatal—This concerns the mother's health before and during pregnancy. Was her nutrition complete and normal? Were there any illnesses related to or that affected the pregnancy? Were any drugs—prescription, over-the-counter, illegal—or alcohol taken during pregnancy? Did the mother smoke? Any complications, such as vaginal bleeding?

- Natal—How difficult or easy was the delivery? Were any analgesics (pain killers) used? Was the child premature or late? By how much? What was the birth order if this was a multiple birth? Did the mother smoke? Any complications, such as breech birth?

- Neonatal—How long was the hospital stay following birth? Were any resuscitation efforts necessary? Were there any initial problems with feeding, breathing, or infections? Any specific illnesses? Were the baby and mother separated after birth? Why and for how long? What was the mother's health after giving birth?

Feeding History

This is also particularly important in the first two years of life, and will need to be addressed if the child is suffering from any digestive disorder or abdominal pain. This is where your records become very important. Your child's needs will be addressed more quickly and more completely if you have this information at your fingertips.

- Infants—Breast-feeding. How long and how frequently does the baby nurse? Do the parents provide any supplements to breast feedings? Any difficulties, such as cracked nipples or a weak suck from the child?

- Infants—Bottle-feeding. What is the type, concentration, and amount of the formula? Be sure to bring the formula in its original packaging. How often is the baby fed, and how much does she take?

- Infants—Digestion. Address difficulties such as regurgitation, colic, and diarrhea.

- Infants—Weaning. How old was the child when he was weaned? What method was used? How was solid food introduced? What was the response? Does the child attempt to feed himself?

- Children—General eating habits. What does she like and dislike? How do the parents address eating problems? Have you kept a diet diary prior to your visit?

Growth and Developmental History

Once again, the first few years are the ones to watch. Then, if problems arise related to slow growth, intellectual development, or behavior, this part of the history will pave the way to a plan. One important note on the developmental history: doctors watch for parents who exaggerate their child's development. You know better than to do that, but the doctor may still assume you are exaggerating the way so many others do. You can show him you are being objective if you give him dates, measurements, and detailed descriptions.

- Physical growth—This will come from the doctor's measurements, but he's mostly watching for weight and height change between visits. If you can provide records that fill out the intervening periods, you may be handing him valuable clues. Watch for slow and rapid changes. Take note of tooth eruption and loss. The doctor is looking for where the child is on the development curve.

- Developmental milestones—The doctor will want to know how old the child was when she achieved these milestones: held up head while lying down, rolled over from back to front and vice versa, sat up with support, sat up by herself, walked with support, walked by herself, said first word, said combinations of words, said sentences, tied shoes by herself, and dressed by herself.

- Sleep—What is the child's sleep pattern? Your records will help. What is the bedtime routine? What type of bed does the child sleep on? Where is it located? Does he have nightmares? How often? Does the child sleep in the parent's bed?

- Toilet training—How has she been toilet trained? How old was she when she started to control her bladder and bowel? Any patterns of bedwetting? Be sure to let the doctor know what terms you use with your child for urination and defecation. This allows her to talk to your child.

- Speech—How large is the child's vocabulary? Does she stutter, hesitate, or continue baby talk? If she had one or the other of these speech patterns and has gotten over it, when did this happen?

- Schooling—Describe the location and environment of the child's nursery or school. How old was he when he started? Has he had any social or academic problems?

Even before your child enters adolescence, your doctor will have to ask him about sex and drugs. These issues are tough on most parents, causing countless hours of worry and conflict. We can't tell you how to work with your child on these issues. Every parent has a unique approach. But every doctor has the same basic approach and the same goal. Sex and drugs can seriously harm children. If your doctor doesn't talk to him, your child is at even greater risk.

As a parent, you have to be sure your doctor asks these questions. You have to be sure your child gives honest answers. Excuse yourself from the room. After you have covered developmental history, tell the doctor that you are leaving so he can ask your child about sex and drugs.

This probably won't put the doctor and your child at ease, but it will force the issue. The issue has to be forced. If your child doesn't learn about the dangers of sex and drugs, he is more likely to fall victim. If his condition is related to sex or drugs and it doesn't come up in the medical history, an appropriate treatment is impossible. No matter how you, as a parent, feel about these issues, you must let the doctor handle the medical side in his own way.

Additional Past Health History

This should come from the parent, but older children can provide details. All of these items are covered for adults as well as children, but they are of particular importance in a pediatric history. As you wrap up the past health history segment, be sure that you have covered the following:

- Childhood illnesses—Be sure to mention if your child has had illnesses like chicken pox, mumps, or measles. Be ready to describe the course of the illness, the treatment, and how it was resolved. It is also very important to mention if the child has been exposed to these illnesses, say through a family member or playmate, even if she didn't get them herself.

- Operations and hospitalizations—Be ready with the name of the hospital, the name of the doctor who performed the operation, and the outcome. If you have those medical records available, bring a copy.

- Accidents and injuries—Even a minor fall or bump that didn't require medical attention at the time could be relevant later. Think about this before the visit. Your doctor may ask.

Current Health: How Are You?

This should come from the parent. If you review the current health section in chapter 3, you will find that most of the questions, tobacco consumption for example, wouldn't apply to most children. We hope. Instead, the current health history for a pediatric exam concentrates on preventive measures. You will want to tell the doctor, of course, about any chronic conditions. If there are none, make sure she knows about immunizations, allergies, and screenings.

Go over the immunization schedule in this chapter before your visit. Check off the ones your child has received. Be sure that you haven't missed any. An exact date is important, since booster programs, which last throughout childhood, have to be followed correctly. Also take careful note of any negative reactions to vaccines. If the child got hives, or got sick soon after for no apparent reason, be sure that your doctor is brought up to date.

Certain allergies are very common to children and infants. Be sure that you call your doctor's attention to any hives, scales, dry or irritated

---

PENICILLIN ALLERGY WARNING SIGNS

Penicillin allergy can be terrifying and dangerous, and there's no way to know if your child has it until it manifests itself. The good news is that it can be treated if caught quickly. Check your child frequently during the seventy-two hours after her first penicillin shot. Any skin eruption should be investigated, especially hives. A more serious sign, which needs immediate action, is swelling in the neck. If not treated, this could prevent the child's breathing. If your child tells you he has trouble swallowing after a penicillin dose, get to a hospital, even if you can't see visual signs of swelling.

skin, or swelling, especially of the sinus and throat. Children can also be hypersensitive to insect bites. If your child is getting his very first dose of penicillin, be sure to tell the doctor that this is the first time.

Current health history for children also includes screening tests. There are quite a few of these, and it's not uncommon for an HMO to miss one. Telling your doctor what tests your child *has* had will prompt him to ask what specific tests he *hasn't* had. It's always a good idea to get this information into the history. Be sure to get your child, at minimum, the following tests from your HMO:

- Hearing
- Hematocrit (tests for the volume of red blood cells in the blood)
- Tuberculosis
- Urinalyses
- Vision

For certain high-risk groups, the following tests are a good idea:

- Sickle cell
- Blood lead
- Cholesterol
- Alpha-antitrypsin deficiency (absence of this blood protein can cause emphysema)

It's the doctor's responsibility to order the right tests, whether the HMO is cutting costs or not. But the list of possible tests is a long one, and tests for high-risk groups are sometimes obscure. It's always a good idea, after you have established what tests the child has had, to ask what other tests he should have. A little comment like "What else should we test for?" or "Have we covered everything?" should do the trick.

How Does Assessment Work for Children?

We've covered the differences between an adult history and a child's history, and given you some tips on how to prepare your child for the exam. But what are the differences in the assessment and decision stages? Do pediatricians use the same methods for assessing and diagnosing kids as regular doctors do for adults?

Almost, but not quite. There are some special considerations for children, but for the most part, you can use the same questions you learned in chapter 3 to get the best assessment and decision for your child. Your doctor runs through the same steps for assessing your child as he does for you: he identifies problems, identifies abnormalities, places abnormalities and problems anatomically, identifies possible processes, creates a hypothesis, tests the hypothesis, and then puts it into words.

But for children, additional questions need to be raised about how the problem affects normal development. These questions should enter the doctor's mind at every stage of his assessment. It's unfortunate that it doesn't always work that way, especially in an HMO.

For one thing, an HMO might not send you to a doctor trained in pediatrics. Since assessment can become so habitual for doctors, he might leave the development question out of his thinking. But even the best-trained family practice doctors can have their thinking affected by HMOs. This brings us back to the idea of "medical necessity."

You will remember how HMOs define medical necessity. It's not a question of what will make the patient better, but what will keep him from getting worse. In the case of a child, his condition may be stable, but it can still affect his development. An HMO might try to get away with the bare minimum of care, treating just the condition without addressing development. This is where you will need to be very alert and ready to fight for your kid.

We saw a case where two parents took their child in for gastrointestinal problems—she wasn't holding down her food, and had constant diarrhea. The HMO treated the problem with the cheapest possible method, and within a month had a patient who could hold down food and seemed to be doing fine. The diarrhea was still there, but didn't seem to be a problem in itself. The parents weren't convinced. They had been measuring and monitoring their child's growth, and saw that it had slowed down considerably.

They showed their records to their doctor and got immediate results. With this additional information added to the history, the doctor asked for an enzyme test. This is an expensive test, just the sort of thing that HMOs want to avoid. But once the parents demonstrated that the child's development was getting worse, even the HMO's own definition of medical necessity couldn't prevent the kid from getting tested. Sure enough, there was an enzyme deficiency. Luckily, it was caught soon enough to be treated.

It is always appropriate to ask your doctor this question: "Will my child's condition affect his development?" This question will force the doctor to reexamine his assessment, to look at the problem from a developmental standpoint. Continue the questioning until you are completely satisfied with the answer. Even if the answer is "no," be sure to ask what you should watch for, what warning signs will let you know if the answer should be "maybe."

Finally, just like you would ask the doctor if it were you on the examining table, ask the doctor "What else could this be?" This is perhaps the most important question an HMO patient can ask. Doctors, just like the rest of us, prefer the most readily available and easiest answer. If it walks like a duck, and sounds like a duck, it's probably a duck. But what if it's a goose? When you ask "What else could this be?" you can inspire the doctor to reconsider his first impression. It's what he's been trained to do.

How Do I Make a Plan for My Child?

You've listened to your doctor's assessment. You've made sure it makes sense. You've thought about whether it accounts for all of your child's symptoms. You've asked how it affects his development, and asked what else it could be. With all your questions and concerns out of the way, you are ready to make a plan.

Work with your doctor to make sure that she knows you are the most important part of your child's treatment team. Be sure that you understand what to watch for, that you know what warning signs mean the treatment isn't working. If medications are involved, be sure you understand what side effects to watch for, and what interactions are possible. If your child needs a medical team, ask the doctor whom you need to recruit.

You are doing the same thing you would do for yourself, but now you are the advocate for your child. We obviously don't need to tell you how important it is to watch your HMO's decision closely; in most cases, though, as long as you are tracking the problem, there's no reason to worry a lot.

Children, it's true, get sicker more quickly than adults. But they also have an amazing ability to bounce back. Their bodies are constantly gearing up for the next growth spurt. Most infections and injuries that get in the way don't stand a chance. Keep this in mind as you reach the decision stage with your doctor.

Your child might not need powerful drugs, even if the condition looks serious. He probably won't need invasive procedures to fix an injury. It's always better to let a child's developing body do most of the work, if possible. Think of your child's development as a steady upward curve. If an injury or infection knocks him off that curve, the best plan is to simply put him back on track and allow nature to take its course.

So consider this as you evaluate the plan. It might sound like the HMO isn't doing enough. You may remember a time when you had similar symptoms and got a more aggressive treatment. But if you take into account the reserves of strength your child has, you may decide that doing less will serve your child better.

What Have I Accomplished?

It seems like a lot of work, guarding your child's health as well as your own against the HMO's cost-cutting practices. But keeping the right records, working with your child to prepare for the visit, and using HEAD to get to the right decision are all things that become easier with practice. And the rewards are outstanding.

Unless you or she becomes very wealthy, your child will grow up in a managed care environment. Her children will be born in a managed care hospital. When you make your HMO safe for your child, you are giving her skills that she will use for the rest of her life, skills she will pass on to your grandchildren. And as your child watches you advocate for her, she is learning about something she may one day do for you.

The next chapter will explain how seniors can navigate managed care and Medicare at the same time. Even if you are young and healthy, read this chapter. You may one day have to be an advocate for an elderly parent. You may one day have to ask someone to advocate for you.

IMMUNIZATION SCHEDULES

Childhood

The following vaccinations are needed by age two. They can be completed in four to five visits to a doctor or clinic.

4 vaccinations	Diphtheria, tetanus, and pertussis (DTP)
3 vaccinations	Polio (IPV or OPV). Note: IPV is now the preferred form
1 vaccination	Measles, mumps, and rubella (MMR)
3–4 vaccinations	Hib (influenza)
3 vaccinations	Hepatitis B (Hep B)
1 vaccination	Varicella (chicken pox)

More than one immunization can be given at the same time as long as they are given in different places in the arms and legs. Children should not get immunizations while they are very sick.

Adolescence

By age thirteen, this series of shots and boosters should be complete:

5 vaccinations	Diphtheria, tetanus, pertussis (DTP or DTaP)
4 vaccinations	Polio (OPV or IPV). Note: IPV is now the preferred form.
2 vaccinations	Measles, mumps, rubella (MMR)
1 vaccination	Varicella (chicken pox)—only if the child has not yet had chicken pox.

Adult

While you are taking care of your child's immunizations, take care of yourself as well. Unfortunately, adults are often lax on receiving their immunizations, but it's as important for adults as it is for kids.

Chicken pox (VZV)	Needed only if you have not had chicken pox.

IMMUNIZATION SCHEDULES (continued)

Adult (continued)

Hepatitis B (Hep B)	Many adults never got the more recently developed Hep B vaccine. If you are one of them, you need this series of three shots immediately.
Influenza (flu)	Even if you are healthy, a yearly flu shot can keep you from spreading the flu to others.
Second MMR	A lot of adults ages twenty-five to thirty-five never got a second MMR shot. If you haven't, talk to your doctor.
Pneumococcal (pneumonia)	All adults over sixty-five and adults any age with chronic conditions like diabetes, lung disease, or kidney disease need this shot.
Tetanus, diphtheria (Td) booster	Needed once every ten years.

Special

If you are traveling (even taking a cruise), be sure to get the following for yourself and your child. These are the immunizations most often missed, even by the most responsible patients. You should start your immunization schedule at least three months before you depart.

Hepatitis A (2 shots)

Meningitis (I shot)

Typhoid fever (lasts for 3 years)

Yellow fever (lasts for 10 years)

~ 9 ~

Getting Great Care over 65

QUESTIONS THIS CHAPTER ANSWERS

◆ How do Medicare HMOs work?

◆ What are the benefits and drawbacks to Medicare HMOs?

◆ How can HEAD and prevention help?

◆ How do I appeal my case?

◆ How do I appeal denied medication?

◆ Why have I been pushed into (or out of) a nursing home?

◆ When should I switch plans?

◆ How will my HMO handle end-of-life decisions?

To many Medicare recipients, it looked like a no-brainer. The government allowed HMOs to sign Medicare contracts, and HMOs started making promises to our seniors—"free" medication, "free" eyeglasses, low monthly payments for 100 percent coverage. It sounded too good to be true. Many seniors found out that it was.

One senior we talked to found this out almost immediately. "The first thing that happened was that they kept putting me off," he told us. "I had to wait nine weeks to get an appointment with my primary care doctor. Then I barely have a chance to get comfortable in his office before he rushes me out the door. I left with a handful of referrals for lab work, and electrocardiogram, and a chest X ray. He didn't even want to give me the chest X ray—I had to insist."

This elderly patient's troubles weren't over yet: "When I started calling around, I found out that I had to travel to four different locations over three days to get all the tests done. I still have my driver's license, but I don't feel comfortable behind the wheel. So do I take a chance in rush hour traffic, or do I take a chance with my health? I took a chance with traffic. I used to get all this done in my doctor's office."

There was an irregularity in the electrocardiogram, and the now-frustrated patient had to go back to his primary care physician to make a plan. "This doctor was much nicer this time, but I guess even he hasn't figured out this managed care thing. He wrote me a prescription that would lower my blood pressure, but when I tried to fill it (and I had to drive way out to a pharmacy that was on the HMO's list), they tell me that the HMO doesn't pay for that drug. So I had to pay the entire cost myself. I told my doctor about it, and he's pretty much 'Well, that's the breaks.' What happened to my free medications? Was my health plan just lying about that? And what if I get sick? Will they still expect me to run all over town to get well?"

This experience sums up what so many seniors are finding out about managed care. Drugs are covered, but not all drugs. The rates are cheaper, but the inconvenience is higher. A ten-minute office visit isn't enough time to get through multiple complaints. And there's a dark cloud on the horizon for many seniors—if they suffer a serious condition, they feel, their HMO will leave them stranded.

There is hope. You can work with your HMO to put a shine on your golden years. All of the methods and advice we have given in the previous chapters will work for seniors as well as for the young and healthy. Using HEAD, following your preventive plan, doing your research, and knowing how to appeal based on medical necessity will help you manage your managed care plan. But we also know that seniors have special needs and concerns. That's why we've devoted this chapter to you.

In this chapter, you will learn about what's wrong with Medicare HMOs, but also what's right. We will show how HEAD and prevention can help. We will give you guidelines for your appeal, and pointers on when to give up and change plans. Finally, and this is unpleasant but very important, we will discuss how to make your HMO a partner in your end-of-life decisions.

Every senior has two needs from his health plan—to save money and to get the best care. It's not easy, but any senior armed with the right information can do both.

What's Wrong with Medicare HMOs?

It's an inescapable fact—there are ways in which managed care is simply incompatible with elder care. HMOs always make more money covering young, healthy suburbanites. An elderly patient with one or more chronic conditions can quickly become a downward drag on an HMO's bottom line. There is no way a profit-minded managed care plan would insure a senior if it weren't for Medicare.

In 1982, during a time of deregulation and budget cuts, the federal government authorized HMOs to get into the Medicare business. The first Medicare HMOs started operation in 1985. They got off to a shaky start. Plans entered the senior market and left within a few years after finding that they just couldn't make money from seniors, even when the government was picking up most of the tab. But in the early nineties, new players began to think that they could learn from the early failures. Federal money always looks good from a distance.

In 1992, only 2.3 million Medicare recipients were in HMOs. In 1999, there were 6.8 million. Why would so many plans go after this high-risk demographic group? One fact explains it all: 80 percent of seniors in Medicare HMOs reside within only ten counties. Those ten counties got the highest reimbursements from the federal government. That's right—where you live makes a huge difference in what kind of care you get.

Let's take a look at how a Medicare HMO is paid. The organization enters into a contract with the Health Care Financing Administration (HCFA). The most typical arrangement is a "risk contract." The HCFA pays the health plan a certain amount for each Medicare recipient, just like an employer would pay a managed care plan a per capita amount for each employee.

But that amount can change drastically depending on where you live. The HCFA looks at historical figures to set rates, and they're based on how much they spent per capita under the old system in your county. Seniors in urban areas have always spent more Medicare money than seniors in rural areas. No one is really sure why, but the result is that Medicare HMOs in cities get more from the government per patient than HMOs in the country.

So if you live in one of these highly compensated areas, you can expect your HMO to roll out the red carpet for you. In Allegheny County, Pennsylvania, plans received an average of nearly $7,500 per senior per year, compared to $4,500 in "poorly compensated" areas. The result: more choice, lower payments, and better treatment. Pittsburgh boasted nine Medicare HMO plans in 1999, all competing with each other on rates and services. Some plans even waived the standard monthly payment for seniors. The most expensive offered coverage at only $43 per month.

The government promises that all this is about to change. Instead of basing Medicare payments to HMOs on location, age, and gender, they will "risk adjust" payments, basing per capita payments on the average total cost of care for individuals who had the same diagnoses in the previous year. So if you are on Medicare and have diabetes, your plan will receive a payment based on how much it costs to treat diabetes, not just on where you live and how old you are.

The idea is to take away some of the risk for managed care plans. Under the demographic-based payments, the HMO would get the same amount whether you were healthy or had diabetes. But as risk adjustment takes effect, they will get more if you have diabetes. That cushions the risk for managed care, but it doesn't take it away completely.

For example, elderly people with diabetes have a greater chance of developing osteoporosis. So even if your plan has been covered to treat your diabetes, they may be wary of giving you the most expensive treatment, assuming that they will need cash reserves to treat broken bones. The risk has been adjusted more appropriately, but it hasn't been eliminated.

This risk can be passed on to you. Your health plan is prepaid by the HCFA for treating any problem you have or may develop. If you started the year healthy, but get sick halfway through, the HMO loses money. If this happens to a large number of their Medicare patients, the HMO goes broke. If you want to assume that the HMO has a really sinister plan, think about how much money they can save if they get paid for treating your diabetes, but then skimp on your treatment. To them, such a strategy would just be good business.

The HCFA is on the right track, but the changes won't be fully in effect until 2004. Even then, you can't count on the government to watch your back. After all, everyone knows that Medicare is headed for bankruptcy eventually, so the HCFA has something in common with managed care. They both want to save money.

Another way they are trying to do this is with "competitive pricing." Experiments are already under way that involve plans bidding for Medicare contracts, just like they do for employers and unions. This will certainly save money, but unless the HMOs and the HCFA alike are as diligent about quality as they are about savings, competitive pricing will force patients to accept a stripped-down, poorly managed, and dangerously low standard of care.

The final years of our lives are expensive. Seniors need more attention, better screening, and more expensive treatments than younger patients. The stakes are higher, and the mistakes are more serious. If you chose a Medicare HMO, you will save money. But you will have to become more aware about your health, better at your research, and more committed to prevention than ever before.

What's Right with Medicare HMOs?

If you can make this system work, however, you can get even better care than you would have in the old fee-for-service Medicare world. The special needs of elders call out for consistent and compassionate management of a comprehensive health program. That's just what managed care can deliver, if you have the right plan and work it in the right way.

When seniors were paying a fee for each service, each visit was more or less a self-contained event. There was no incentive to promote a holistic approach. Since many seniors see several specialists for several different conditions, those self-contained events could create some pretty nasty side effects.

Take medication for example. A seventy-year-old man might be taking ten different medications prescribed by five different specialists. None of these fee-for-service specialists have discussed this patient with each other. None of them knows what the other is doing. The patient is being thoroughly overmedicated, and no one has a clue. He reports dizziness to his neurologist, who writes out a prescription for yet another medication, which interacts with his blood pressure medication that he got from his cardiologist. The next day he collapses on the golf course and is rushed to the hospital.

Twenty percent of Medicare patient hospitalizations are directly caused by failure to follow medication programs or adverse drug interactions. That means hundreds of millions of dollars every year are drained from the Medicare trust fund by easily preventable problems. Precious time is stolen from the last years of our senior's lives. And let us not forget that once in the hospital, seniors are particularly susceptible to infections and procedural complications.

An HMO has a clear financial incentive to keep you out of the hospital. If they can cut hospitalization by one-fifth among their Medicare population just by making sure their patients take their medications and watching out for drug interactions, believe us, they will do it. And they are ready to do it. The best managed care organizations specialize in coordinated services. The team members are there, ready to work together, ready to communicate, ready to keep their hospitalization rates down. All they need is your complete information.

Medicare was set up over three decades ago and has very slowly adapted to the lessons of preventive medicine. It was never intended to treat chronic problems over a long period of time, only to cure acute conditions. But seniors, even those with chronic conditions, are living much longer these days than they did in the 1960s.

The massive baby boom transition into retirement will coincide with an increase in the average life span. Today, seniors account for about 13 percent of the population, and 36 percent of all health care expenditures. By 2030, seniors will account for 36 percent of the population. Ten million baby boomers will celebrate their ninetieth birthdays, and one million will live to see their one hundredth. Fee-for-service Medicare was not built to treat this long-lived generation.

That means the torch will pass to the HMOs. They are equipped to maintain health, to treat problems over time, and to work on prevention. They also have a financial incentive to do so. We can see this happening in many small ways that don't cost the HMO much money, but save seniors from expensive and invasive surgery and ultimately save lives.

One plan gives free shower chairs to its elderly patients who need them. Another advertises that it will provide free transportation to its clinic three times a month. Several plans are offering free seminars, led by doctors, devoted to education about cholesterol, hypertension, and other problems that affect the elderly. These are small things that can make a huge difference.

If shower chairs save three seniors in a given plan from needing hip replacements, that saves the plan tens of thousands of dollars. If a cholesterol seminar changes the habits of just one attendee, he might not need a $14,000 angiogram to check for coronary artery disease. And if transportation ensures that patients get to their appointments, simple problems can be solved before they become major. These are win-win solutions for the patient and the plan.

HMOs are learning about how to care for seniors, but they still have a way to go. Government regulation will help. Creative solutions will help. But when it comes to your individual needs, only you can provide the kick that reminds managed care what it has to do.

How Can HEAD and Prevention Help?

Some doctors, we are sorry to say, hold onto a stereotype of their senior patients. You've seen this stereotype played out in movies and television shows—the ever-complaining elder. He doesn't have a chief complaint, but comes in with a long list of unrelated grievances, thankful for the chance to express them to someone who *has* to listen. If your doctor starts pushing you to limit your complaints before you even start, he's probably thinking you fit into this mold.

But using HEAD, just like we explained in chapter 3, will completely erase this prejudice from his mind. Move quickly to the chief complaint. Make sure it's a succinct statement. Then give him the history of your present illness using the seven parts of the symptom we outlined in chapter 3: location, quality, quantity or severity, timing, setting, aggravating and relieving factors, and associated symptoms.

It's when you get to associated symptoms that you will want to slow down. Seniors often have multiple symptoms. How can you tell if yours are associated with your chief complaint or not? The best way to find out is to ask a direct question. "Doctor, I have a number of other symptoms, and I don't know if they are related to this complaint or not. Can I list them for you?" She will say, "Of course." Then you can give your list: "I am also constipated. Is this relevant? I am also suffering from pain in my knee. Is this relevant? I have this slight discoloration on my skin. Is this relevant?" Every time you get a "yes," you can go through the seven parts of that symptom with your doctor. That way, you can be sure that each symptom you experience enters into her thought process.

We know it's harder to use HEAD when you have two or more chief complaints. But the solution is simple. Discuss them separately. Say the doctor asks you, "What seems to be the problem?" Reply, "I have two complaints." Then give the doctor the one that is most important to you. After you have finished with the history of the present illness, go back and use HEAD again for the second complaint. Remember your goals: (1) Get the information out on the table; (2) Keep your thoughts organized; (3) Get the doctor on your side.

When you come in for a screening test, we understand that it's tempting to bring up other problems. Why shouldn't you? You are in the office, you have a doctor at your disposal. But that doctor has a long line of patients waiting to see him. If he doesn't get through his day, some administrator upstairs will notice. But you don't want to ignore a complaint just because he's on the clock.

So think about what problems you have before your screening appointment. Make a call to your HMO and explain that in addition to your screening, you would like to discuss a separate problem: "Will the doctor I am seeing for the test be able to help? If not, can I get an appointment on the same day to address this problem?" If the problem pops into your mind while you are in the doctor's office, ask in the same way: "I know you are busy, but I have an additional concern that needs attention. Can we discuss this now, or can I see you later today? This will only take a minute." Since you know HEAD, you are being perfectly honest when you say it will only take a minute.

Now back to your history. All the segments of your history that we gave in chapter 3 are important. But when you are over sixty-five, you want to pay special attention to your family history. Traits that led to problems your parents experienced in their retirement years may have been passed on to you. The conditions they cause might not appear until you have reached the same stage of life. You may have brought these issues up when you were in middle age. You may have put them on the form you filled out in the waiting room. Still it's important to frequently remind your doctor what problems your parents had. Each condition you raise should lead to a preventive plan. You want to know what tests can catch the problem early on. You want to know what lifestyle changes you should make. And you want to know what education or information your HMO can offer.

As a senior, the other part of your history that's especially important is your current medication list. As we mentioned above, seniors are hospitalized at an alarming rate for adverse drug interactions. Before each visit, empty out your medicine cabinet. Bring even the drugs you aren't taking right now. Having the actual bottles will help you immeasurably. If your doctor notices a drug that you shouldn't be taking, he can toss it in the trash right away. That means you won't have a chance to forget his directions once you leave the office. Managing several different courses of medication can be difficult for anyone. It's easy to get confused.

HEAD can push aside your doctor's prejudices, win her over to your side, and lead directly to a comprehensive treatment plan. We recommend it for any patient, any age. But we also realize that as patients get older, they can have greater difficulty summoning the focus required to use it effectively. As you move through your golden years, consider finding an advocate.

Your advocate can be a friend or relative, anyone who can take the time to come with you to your most important appointments. Even if you know that your cognitive skills are still sharp, having an advocate in the room is important. You need to have a backup team captain who knows something about your medical history. If you ever become incapacitated, knowing that a loyal advocate can take over will give you and your doctor peace of mind.

These few tips should get you through the history with flying colors. Now we have a few additional tips about prevention. Revisit chapter 5, which outlines the major preventive measures appropriate to your age group, habits, and family history, and chapter 6, which explains how to build a team. As an elderly patient, you will need, more than ever, to build a team devoted to prevention. You will need to see specialists before problems arise.

HMOs should be ready and willing to help keep you from getting sick. After all, they will save money later if they spend a little on you now, as long as you stay with the plan to reaps the benefits of this prevention. The best Medicare HMOs will do this without your insistence, but sadly, many HMOs fall short. You may need to gather your resources—information, advocates, and your primary care doctor.

Medicare HMOs are required by contract to provide the same quality of care that Medicare patients would receive under fee-for-service. But quality is difficult to measure. HMOs are receiving 5 percent less than the average cost of treating patients under Medicare fee-for-service. They are required to provide the screening test you need, but they might not make it easy for you.

There are a few first steps toward getting preventive treatments. First, understand what you need. Review chapter 5 and discuss it with your primary care doctor. Make sure your doctor knows your family history and your concerns. Get your doctor on your side. See to it that he has good reasons to recommend the treatment, and that he puts these reasons in your chart.

If these first steps fall short, if the preventive treatment you need is still denied, it's time to appeal.

How Do I Appeal My Case?

Uncle Sam has removed much of the guesswork from the appeals process for Medicare patients. A private HMO patient has to live with the appeals process set up by his health plan and, in some cases, regulated by the state. But Medicare HMO patients who want to appeal follow a standard process that doesn't vary from plan to plan or state to state. Don't let your HMO tell you otherwise. The law says they all have to play by the government's rules.

When you are ready to appeal, place a call to the Medicare help line at (800) MEDICAR. Ask the service representative who answers what the first step should be. We are advising you to place this call because regulations may change; you want to have everything in order the first time you go to bat. When it is time to write an appeal letter to your HMO, use the template on page 184. Once your appeal is set in motion, you can expect to go through these stages:

- You may be entitled to an "expedited decision." Medicare HMOs are required to decide on appeals in seventy-two hours if your life, health, or ability to return to "maximum function" is in jeopardy. This is especially important to know if your treatment has been stopped or if you have been discharged from a hospital or nursing home. Try to make a case for an expedited decision. If it sounds reasonable, the HMO is unlikely to decline.

- Notice to the member. The managed care organization must let you know that they have received your appeal. This is also the point where you learn if you will receive an expedited decision. If you don't get an expedited decision, your HMO has sixty days to respond.

- Determination by the managed care organization. This is your HMO's first chance to review its decision. This will be based on the medical records it has available.

- Reconsideration by managed care organization. If the determination does not go in your favor, you have the right to reconsideration. You can present any new information that will bolster your case, either in writing or in person. If your appeal is over a very expensive procedure, consider hiring an attorney to present your case for you. If not an attorney, consider an advocate, such as a family member or sympathetic doctor.

- Reconsideration by outside review. A denied case that demands further appeal will now be sent to the HCFA, which will send it to the Center for Health Dispute Resolution (CHDR), contracted by the HCFA to handle all its appeals. Know that an independent review doesn't automatically mean a patient-centered bias. In 1996, the CHDR upheld the managed care's decision in 65.5 percent of the cases it heard.

- Hearing before an administrative law judge (ALJ), if the claim is over $100. These judges are hard to get to. Their schedules are full, and it may take up to a year to get a hearing. Once you are there, you should keep in mind that these judges oversee all Social Security matters, not just health care. They may not know all the ins and outs of Medicare.

- Review by the Department Appeals Board. The next rung on this long ladder is the Health and Human Services' Department Appeals Board. Again, you may have a long wait, and since you are getting even further from Medicare, you will have to be crystal clear about your request.

- Judicial review. The very last hope is to bring your case to federal court. This stage is only available to you if the amount concerned is over $1,000. Very few cases get to this level, which in any event may only be reached years after the original appeal was filed.

Few seniors will want to wait that long to see their case resolved. The good news is that if you are on Medicare, you don't have to. At almost any time, you have the right to switch out of your managed care plan and into another, or back to traditional Medicare. You may forfeit some extras and other benefits, but the 80 percent coverage granted by Medicare cannot be denied to you. We will talk about switching in the next section.

How Do I Appeal Denied Medication?

Since traditional Medicare doesn't cover medication, HMOs have quite a bit of leeway in deciding which drugs are covered and which ones aren't. The marketing literature seniors get from managed care plans make it sound like prescriptions are free, and that makes their offers hard to turn down. Once inside, however, Medicare patients feel like the free prescriptions deal was simply bait to lure them into a trap.

Each HMO has a "formulary," a list of approved drugs. Anything that's not on this list you have to pay for out of pocket. That's important to remember when you are signing up for a plan. If you are on medications, be sure that the ones you know you need are on your plan's formulary.

If you are denied a medication that your doctor recommends, your only course is to appeal the denial based on medical necessity. The HMO can't turn you down if you can prove that your condition will get worse without the drug. However, appeals for medication don't go through the HCFA procedures for appeals. You have to go through the HMO's own appeals process.

Remember that what's "medically necessary" isn't what makes you better. It's what keeps you from getting worse. That's why HMOs had such an easy time turning down Viagra prescriptions. Certainly their patients lives would be better with the prescription, but if they don't get it, they won't get worse. You need to be able to pinpoint exactly how your condition is deteriorating because you haven't gotten a particular drug. The best ally in this struggle is, again, your own doctor.

Why Have I Been Pushed Into (or Out of) a Nursing Home?

It's because of money. HMOs institutionalize their patients because of money. You don't have to go, but if you need around-the-clock medical care following a debilitating illness or stroke, a nursing home will be on your treatment plan.

It doesn't make a lot of sense unless you count the money. Medicare also won't cover long-term stays in a skilled nursing facility, only short stays for recovery. Managed care plans cover more days at 100 percent coverage, but that means they will work harder to keep your stay short. They can legally do this because skilled nursing home care often produces ambiguous results. The stay doesn't cure you, it just provides a safe place for the treatment to take effect.

One example of how lax managed care can be about managing recovery from debilitating illness can be found in a recent study of post-stroke patients. Patients who recovered at a skilled nursing home facility were compared to patients who received care at a rehabilitation facility, where they were put on a program of light physical and mental exercise. The rehabilitation patients, unsurprisingly, were better able to function day-to-day than those who were simply monitored in a skilled nursing home. But still, most HMOs guide patients to skilled nursing facilities—the cheaper option. Why? Because the study found no difference in the rate of second strokes between the two groups. Here again, the HMO's emphasis is on keeping you from getting worse, not toward making you better or improving your quality of life.

That doesn't mean you can't make a case for rehabilitation as opposed to institutional care. You just have to phrase it in the HMO's own terms. Discuss your options with your doctor and try to apply them to your own life. Point to specific activities that you need to perform, such as shopping for food, driving, or volunteer work. Use the phrase "maximum functionality." It's a phrase that the HCFA uses to judge cases. If your doctor thinks that rehabilitation has a better chance of returning you to maximum functionality than institutional care, you have a case.

Whether you are in an institution for your recovery or receiving care at home, you may have to appeal when your benefit runs out. Traditional Medicare Part A covers the first twenty days of your stay in a skilled nursing facility at no cost to you. After that, you pay $96 a day up to one hundred days. After that, your coverage runs out. Medicare HMOs offer one hundred days, if medically necessary, at no additional charge. Sounds good, until you find that a bean counter in the utilization review department decides you have stayed long enough.

We know that you want to get out of the nursing care facility as soon as possible—and you should. But how soon is too soon? There are a few questions you need to ask yourself before you allow yourself to be sent packing:

- Have your treatment goals been met? You should be clear on your goals before you enter the nursing facility. Can you be sure the treatment has accomplished all of them?

- Can you feed, dress, and clean yourself? If you can't, your HMO has no business moving you out on your own.

- Are you steady on your feet? Can you get around? There's no excuse for sending you home if you are liable to injure yourself from a fall once you are there. It shouldn't make sense to the HMO either. After all, they will have to pay if you take a spill.

- Do you believe your condition will get worse if you don't get constant care? This question is more important than all the others. It's the one that will push your appeal through.

Federal law protects patients in nursing homes from rapid eviction. Any appeal you make must be put on a fast track—the above mentioned "expedited decision" that gets you an answer in seventy-two hours. And recent federal law prohibits a nursing facility that pulls out of the Medicare program from evicting its Medicare patients. There's also a strong movement to reform the nation's nursing homes, one-quarter of which have been cited for "violations that threaten the safety of residents," according to the General Accounting Office. But that shouldn't cause you to let down your guard, whether you are entering a nursing home or being told to leave one.

A final word of caution on skilled nursing facilities. Neither Medicare nor managed care will pay for long-term "custodial care." Both systems only admit patients to nursing homes for recovery from specific acute illnesses. Very few patients realize this until it is too late. A recent survey of baby boomers by the American Health Care Association found that only 6 percent carry coverage for long-term care. Sixty-eight percent know they are not ready to pay for a nursing home. This is a disaster waiting to happen.

If long-term nursing care is covered neither by Medicare nor by managed care, who does cover it? Companies offering separate insurance packages for just this area of need. These can be very expensive, depending on how young and healthy you are when you start paying for coverage. The alternative? Pay the nursing home out of pocket, which costs on average $40,000 per year, but as high as $100,000 per year in some areas. Do this for a little while, and you will be so poor that you will be eligible for Medicaid. That's a very real option, one that many have used as a last resort.

Start early, plan ahead. You can't wait until you need long-term care before you apply for the insurance. If you buy the policy when you are fifty-five and healthy, you can pay as little as $500 per year and be covered for four years of care. But if you wait until you are seventy, the same policy will cost over $2,700 per year. Talk to your adult children about the costs of this additional and expensive insurance and see if they can help. After all, they are investing in their inheritance.

When Should I Switch?

Age has its privileges. While you might be bounced around by the bureaucracies of the government on one side and your HMO on the other, you always have an escape hatch. You can leave your managed care plan at any time without losing full coverage. If you start an appeal and the long waits and paper shuffling don't agree with you, you can just walk away to get the coverage you need.

In some cases you won't even have to walk very far. Many HMOs in key states are changing to "Medicare + Choice," an initiative that expands the options for Medicare patients. Plans that participate in this program can offer seniors coverage on a variety of models. This means if you are frustrated with the limits of your strict network, you can add a point of service option to your basic coverage, allowing you to go outside the network for a higher co-payment.

You can also leave managed care altogether. If you are in your first twelve months of enrollment with a Medicare HMO, you can leave the plan at any time and revert to your Medigap policy, if it's still available. Whether you leave your plan for another managed care organization or leave managed care altogether, all it takes is a letter to your HMO stating that you have dropped the plan. The change takes effect on the first day of the next month, and your Medicare benefits kick in automatically.

Consider this course if you need a short-term and affordable treatment that basic Medicare will cover but your HMO won't. Once you get your treatment from a fee-for-service doctor, you can always go back to managed care. Say you would prefer to recover from a debilitating illness at home rather than in a nursing facility. Most HMOs will only cover home care if it's preapproved and deemed medically necessary. If you are denied, check to see if you meet Medicare's conditions for home care. If you do, home care will cost nothing to you under traditional Medicare. You will have to pay 20 percent of the costs of durable medical equipment, like wheelchairs, hospital beds, or walking aids, but the service is free.

Convincing a fee-for-service doctor that you need home care, or any other treatment, will be much easier than convincing the HMO's utilization review doctors. A fee-for-service doctor can spend as much Medicare money as he wants, as long as he deems it medically necessary—and he's using his own definition of that term. The HMO doctors are under intense pressure *not* to spend money, and have to work with the HMO's definition of the term.

Fee-for-service doctors used to stay away from Medicare patients whenever possible. The government rates were much less than the rates of the indemnity insurers. These days, Medicare patients are the best payers in town. There are hardly any indemnity patients left. If you leave your managed care plan to have a specific treatment handled, you will find fee-for-service doctors fighting each other to get that Medicare money.

You may want to switch out of your plan to have a specific problem treated, or you may have a general problem with the way your HMO conducts business. You shouldn't make the decision to drop a plan lightly, but you should keep your HMO aware, especially during appeals, that you have the power to walk. Take another look at the warning signs we gave in chapter 4. If your HMO exhibits any of these practices, take a hard look at your options. For seniors, we should add and emphasize the following warning signs:

- Changing rules. A health maintenance organization can, at any time, decide a medication or treatment is ineffective and drop it from its list. If you are benefiting from a certain treatment, it shouldn't be taken away. Appeal, and if it doesn't look like you are getting results, find out who will cover your treatment.

- Readmittance for chronic conditions. If you are constantly returning to the hospital for treatment of the same condition, the HMO isn't doing its job. The plan isn't even looking out for its own bottom line. Research your condition thoroughly. Find out what the readmittance rate *should* be. When you go shopping among different plans, find out how each would deal with your problem. Remember that no Medicare HMO can turn you away, no matter how sick you are.

- Doctor warning signs. Some doctors just won't let go of their prejudices toward the elderly. If your doctor treats you like a child even after you have used HEAD, cooperated in forming a plan, and done your best to follow it, change doctors or change plans.

- Fraud and abuse. Medicare fraud hurts us all. It can also be dangerous to your health. Any doctor that falsifies records to get a higher payment has entered dangerous information into your chart. Watch for unreasonable billing, billing for services not provided, evidence of kickbacks, or separate charges for services that should be included in a single service. Report your suspicions to the Inspector General's office at (800) HHS-TIPS. Start shopping.

Even if you are perfectly happy with your plan, you may be forced to shop around. Medicare HMOs have a chance to withdraw from the program every year. In 1998, as the entire managed care industry slumped, 360,000 seniors nationwide received letters informing them that their HMOs would no longer insure Medicare patients. The worst part of it was that the areas affected were the ones where seniors had the least choice. Managing elder care is a risky business, and when a plan starts to dip into the red, it's usually the first program to be dropped.

You can't stop your HMO from dropping you and your peers, but you can stay informed. When a plan decides to pull out of the program, it must inform the HCFA ninety days before the end of the year. Letters must go out to members sixty days before the end of the year. A public notice in a newspaper must appear thirty days before the end of the year. Coverage for Medicare patients terminates on January 1, and those who haven't found new HMOs automatically revert to traditional Medicare. If you make a habit of checking on your HMO's status each year in October, you can buy yourself an extra thirty days to shop for a new plan, get that test or treatment you've been putting off, and stock up on your prescriptions.

Shopping for a new plan can be easier for seniors than it is for the average consumer. For one thing, there are fewer plans to choose from. And the HCFA has developed a terrific, easy-to-use database of the HCFA's Medicare HMO in the nation. Every senior in managed care should look at the HCFA's "Medicare Compare" service at www.medicare.gov. Once you enter your region and your special needs, you will get a table of side-by-side comparisons of services, costs, and quality indicators. Don't stop there. Check your data from the HCFA by calling the prospective plan. Look for information specific to your needs:

- Be sure your drugs are covered.

- Be sure the plan's pharmacies are convenient.

- Be sure the plan has a case management program for your specific conditions.

- Be sure the plan has been in the program for a long time. Plans new to Medicare generally should be avoided.

- Look for plans that offer creative solutions to the special problems of seniors, like free transportation, free seminars, and help with accident prevention.

You should never feel helpless in your Medicare HMO. There are rules it must follow, and services it must provide. The ability to switch at any time, however, is the most powerful protection that seniors have against HMO cost- and corner-cutting. When you are faced with an appeal, a bureaucratic mix-up, or a rude doctor, remind yourself that you don't have to stand for it. You can walk, and you can take your Medicare money with you.

End-of-Life Decisions: Will My HMO Kill Me?

None of us like the idea of a time when we won't be able to make our own decisions about how we will be treated or not treated for a life-threatening illness. We push the possibility out of our minds. When we do so, we leave our family members an impossible question if this difficult situation ever comes to pass. If we don't tell someone what we want in advance, all they can do is guess. And they may never know if they got it right.

Now throw the economic realities of managed care into the mix. A doctor can explain a patient's situation and chances for survival in many different ways, subtly influencing family members' decisions. A fee-for-service doctor makes money for his hospital if he keeps his patient alive. An HMO doctor saves money for his organization if he lets the patient die.

An eighty-five-year-old woman is admitted to the hospital. She's already had one hip replacement, and one heart bypass. Now she's back in the hospital because she aspirated food into her lung and has pneumonia. She was briefly conscious an hour ago, but incoherent. Now she's unconscious and her condition is getting worse. The doctor gets the family together for the most serious decision of their lives. Should this patient be classified as "do not resuscitate" (DNR) or not?

A doctor could tell the family, "There's a good chance that tonight or tomorrow her oxygenation will fall. If she's DNR, she will pass away. If she's full code, or full resuscitation, we'll give her CPR, put her on a breathing machine, give her medications, and she will live. She might even bounce back and live a full life for a few months. What do you want to do?"

Or a doctor could tell the family, "Tonight or tomorrow, her oxygenation will fall. If she's DNR, we can make her comfortable and she will pass away. Or we could pound on her chest, cut a hole in her throat for an artificial breathing tube, put her on medications to keep her failing heart beating, and she will live. But she might stay on the machine indefinitely and never regain consciousness. What do you want to do?" A doctor has the ability to get the answer he wants. It's just a matter of emphasis.

In situations like this, we want to trust our doctors. We want to believe they have our best interests at heart. Most of them do. But even the best can be influenced by their organization's business needs, which have nothing to do with your health. Each day on life support can cost $3,000. This fact should never influence your decision, but a doctor can covertly put that figure into the equation.

The only way to keep your HMO from helping to make the decision for you is to prepare advance directives. Talk to your family about your wishes, and try to be as specific as possible. Make sure your doctor knows your wishes. Have a copy of your advance directives placed in your medical records. Give a copy to a lawyer. Once you have covered these bases, you can be sure that your wishes, and not the HMO's, will be followed.

An advance directive can be in the form of a living will or a durable power of attorney for health care. A living will is a document that spells out what kind of medical care you want or *do not* want should you ever become incapacitated. Many states have standard living will forms, which you can obtain from your state Attorney General's Office or your state Medicare counseling program.

A durable power of attorney for health care authorizes someone else to make medical decisions for you if you are incapacitated. This document is vital if you want someone other than a family member, such as a common-law spouse or same-sex partner, to make the call.

Laws on advance directives vary from state to state. Some states require a living will, some require a durable power of attorney, and some require both. If you frequently travel between two or more states, it's a good idea to make sure you know the laws of each. Many states issue a wallet-sized card that instructs emergency medical services what to do in your case. These are often issued by the state emergency medical services program, and usually have to be signed by your primary care doctor.

You have the right to make these important decisions about your health, but you can only do so if you have advance directives in place before you become incapacitated. You owe it to your loved ones to make their decision more clear. You owe it to yourself to make sure your wishes are carried out. How you will end your life is an intensely personal decision, and you should never leave it to a large, complex organization like an HMO to help your family decide.

What Have I Accomplished?

There are dangers in your later years, and dangers in managed care. But if you use the protections built into the system, you can minimize the risks to your health. With a preventive treatment program in place, you will live longer and have even less need for inconvenient visits to your HMO. When you do get sick, your doctor can be your ally, your research can be your tool, and your ability to leave your plan can be your saving grace when all else fails.

There is a great deal of concern these days about the future of

Medicare. It will certainly be a hot political issue for at least the next decade. There is plenty to be worried about, but this is also an exciting time. Patients, doctors, and administrators are trying out creative solutions that, if successful, will mean that everyone wins. Once you have taken care of your own health, take a look at what is happening to Medicare. Get involved through your community action groups, state boards, and local not-for-profits. Seniors represent a powerful political force. If you can effect a positive change, you can help save Medicare for yourself and your grandchildren.

RESOURCES FOR MEDICARE AND MANAGED CARE

Community Service Society
105 East 22 Street
New York, NY 10010
(212) 614–5401
www.cssny.org
Helps consumers with information on Medicaid and managed care.

Health Care Financing Administration
7500 Security Blvd.
Baltimore, MD 21244
(410) 786-3000
www.hcfa.gov
Government agency that oversees Medicare and Medicaid programs.

National Health Law Program
2639 S. La Cienega Blvd.
Los Angeles, CA 90034
(310) 204–6010
www.healthlaw.org
Advocates for the elderly and disabled, offers training programs.

American Association of Retired Persons
601 E Street, NW
Washington, DC 20049
(800) 424-3410
www.aarp.org
Offers educational publications and training.

Medicare Rights Center
1460 Broadway
New York, NY 10036
(212) 869–3850
Runs an information/help hotline and offers several publications.

~ 10 ~
Managing Your Mental Health Care

QUESTIONS THIS CHAPTER ANSWERS

◆ *How will my HMO treat my mental health?*
◆ *What kind of therapy should I expect?*
◆ *Should I be worried about being medicated?*
◆ *What is a "carved-out" mental health program?*
◆ *How can I use HEAD for psychiatric conditions?*
◆ *How will my teenager's mental health be treated?*
◆ *Will my HMO keep my mental health secrets?*

A fifty-three-year-old man makes his first visit in years to the doctor for a persistent headache. His doctor orders all the appropriate tests and asks the questions that would lead him to a physical cause, but finds nothing wrong. It's probably just one of those things, the doctor decides, and sends the patient off with a prescription for ibuprofen.

Two weeks later, the same patient is back with a different complaint. His lower back has felt tight for a week. One day, when he didn't take the pain killers he was using for his headache, his lower back felt like it was a field of knots. "Try to get some light exercise," the doctor says. "Stay on the pain killers, and if it gets worse, see me for a referral to a chiropractor."

A month later, the patient says he has trouble urinating. Weeks after that, he has sharp stomach pains and can't sleep. He's been so tired he missed work. His doctor continues to put out these brush fires the only way he knows how—with medications and recommendations—but the patient keeps coming back.

HMOs have a not very complimentary word for this patient. He's an "overutilizer," someone who drains money and time from the organization for treatment of minor complaints. In truth, he's probably depressed. All his symptoms, none of which have an apparent physical cause, are most likely symptoms of an underlying mental condition.

In the old days, this patient may have gone to his family doctor for years seeking answers in the wrong place. He may have known his life wasn't exactly as he wanted it to be, but he probably never thought his mental problems were so serious that he needed therapy. No one was out to control costs and cut back on his visits, so the underlying mental problem might have never been caught and addressed.

Managed care companies were never too keen on getting into mental health services. Although psychiatric care has the potential to lower the cost of treating overutilizers like the man above, it can also be a can of very expensive worms. The latest and most effective psychiatric drugs are some of the most costly. A patient can stay in therapy for years and still never feel better. There are dozens of types of therapy, and it's hard to say which one delivers the best results. It's hard to judge who needs mental health services and who doesn't. It's hard to find a yardstick that will measure the quality of any mental health treatment.

But the companies that bought HMO contracts for their employees insisted on mental health services. They could see the benefit, even if the managed care companies couldn't. They could see how workdays were being lost to depression, psychosomatic illness, substance abuse, and personal crises. So employers and managed care companies got together and hammered out the compromise that now affects the mental health of millions of insured patients.

Mental health is the stepchild of the managed care industry. It shouldn't be like that. Half of all adults will use mental health services at some point in their lives. One out of four women and one out of ten men will seek treatment for depression. Many more could benefit from treatment but are discouraged from or intimidated by the idea of going into therapy. Mental health problems like depression, substance abuse, and anxiety are widespread and have a direct impact on society at all levels—at work, at home, in our communities. But managed care remains reluctant to take them on.

The irony of managed care's failure in this area is that treating mental health problems is easier than ever before. The stigma of being in therapy or on medication has all but vanished. The drugs developed over the last ten years to treat mental conditions are just short of miraculous. Concern over the mental health problems of children forced state and local governments to widen and improve access to services, a change that was underway but still incomplete when managed care took over.

So the services and treatments are out there—you just have to convince your HMO to provide them. All of the techniques and tips we have given in previous chapters can easily be adapted to mental health problems. In fact, we believe that mental health problems should be treated no differently from physical problems. They are equally important, and should be given the same degree of attention in any insurance plan. If you can convince your HMO of this fact, you and your family will receive well-rounded coverage that leads to total health, in both body and mind.

In this chapter, we will show you how mental health services have been separated from physical treatment, and how this "carving out" affects you. We will discuss how you should use HEAD to address psychological problems, and what to expect in return. We will also devote a section of this chapter to the mental health problems of teens, who so often fall through the current system's wide cracks. We will then tell you who should be on your mental health team, and finally look at a question with no easy answers—"How confidential are my visits?"

How Will My HMO Treat Mental Health?

Your managed care company would like you to change the way you think about mental health care. You can't expect a bearded psychoanalyst who asks you how you feel about your mother. You can't expect years of therapy covering issues from your toilet training to your last failed relationship. Managed care plans won't provide that. Under their own definition of medically necessary, they don't have to.

Remember, a treatment is medically necessary if denying it will make the patient worse. Since psychotherapy can be a lifelong process, it's hard to prove that it truly prevents the patient from getting worse. A patient who has depression but doesn't get psychotherapy won't necessarily get worse, and may not even get better in a measurable way.

So all managed care has to do is keep you stable. If you are stressed because of a job loss, depressed because of a divorce, or feeling suicidal because of a recent tragedy, a managed care plan that covers mental health services will jump in to treat that problem until you are back to normal. If "normal" for you is still far from happy, you will still be far from happy when your treatment is finished. Managed care health services are set up to treat your specific problems and get you through crises. Long-term psychiatric care is not part of the typical coverage.

This is a real shame, because there are plenty of people in managed care who can benefit from treatment of general conditions like chronic relationship problems or phase-of-life issues. Those people now have to pay out of pocket if they want to battle their personal demons. But it's even worse for the seriously mentally ill—people with incurable but treatable conditions like schizophrenia, bipolar disorder, or major depressive disorder. Their treatments are ongoing and very expensive. New drugs have come to their aid, but few HMOs will include them in their formularies.

Even under traditional indemnity insurance, mental health was an afterthought, accounting for about 8 percent of the premium. When managed care took over, the new plans started looking for places to make cuts, and mental health was an easy place to start. Most managed care companies spend about 3 percent of their revenues on mental health. They've achieved savings in a number of ways—problem-oriented therapy, new medications, and "carving out" mental health services. To help you through this part of the managed care maze, we will first explain what your health plan is up to, and then show you what to watch out for.

What Kind of Therapy Will I Get?

Managed care doesn't care about your feelings. Therapy is expensive, and your HMO isn't about to foot the bill for a therapy session if the therapist is just a passive sounding board for the patient's problems. Managed care plans are interested in getting you through therapy as quickly as possible. They want to see results.

So they've dusted off an old and successful method called "cognitive therapy" to help move you along. This isn't necessarily a bad thing. Cognitive therapy has been practiced for over twenty-five years, and unlike many other therapies, it produces measurable results. The goal of cognitive therapy is to change the way you think, to give you the tools to look at your problems in a new light.

Say a patient tells his therapist that he's depressed. Why? He thinks he's an unlikable person, the world is a hostile place, and his future looks bleak. An "empathic response" therapist would typically say something like "That sounds rough," or "Tell me more about why you think you will never succeed." Each response from the therapist is designed to prompt the patient to dig deeper into his psyche. Somewhere, down there, is a long-hidden cause of the depression.

A cognitive therapist, on the other hand, takes an active role in helping the patient examine his current complaints. The goal is to help the patient see where he has overgeneralized and perceived catastrophe where it doesn't exist. The idea is that a patient is depressed because he has a "negative triad." That means a negative view of himself, a negative view of the world, and a negative view of the future.

So a cognitive therapist might say, "Let's take these one at a time. Let's look at whether you are a likable person. You told me earlier that you volunteer at the animal shelter each week. You also told me you helped your daughter build her first-prize science fair project. It certainly looks as if you are likable. There may be parts of your personality that are unlikable, but other parts are very kind." The therapist isn't just doing this exercise to make the patient feel better. If the therapist succeeds, the patient will be able to actually change his way of thinking.

This is a very brief and incomplete description of a complicated process, but it is what you should expect from managed mental health care. There are several reasons HMOs favor cognitive therapy. First, for mild to moderate depression, this therapy has a relatively high rate of success. Second, it's time-limited. Patients are encouraged and prepared to move on. Third, nondoctors can do it. The training is intense, but nurse practitioners, physician assistants, and social workers can be taught to work with patients using this model.

But this therapy also has its limitations. Severely depressed patients need substantial time in therapy and sufficient medication if this technique is to help. In cases where there really is a deeply buried problem causing the depression, cognitive therapy will fall short. But for what HMOs typically treat—specific problems and crises—cognitive therapy is a great choice. The patient can get on with her life, and the managed care company can save money.

Should I Be Worried about Being Medicated?

There's a lot of talk these days about how managed care companies are over-medicating their mental health patients. To some, it might seem like HMOs are just trying to avoid expensive therapy in favor of drugs. Critics charge that these medications don't treat the underlying problem—that they are just Band-Aids for the mind.

In fact, the antidepressants Prozac, Paxil, and Zoloft are among the ten most-prescribed medications in this country. Their popularity was already assured before managed care became the standard of care that it is today. But the question remains: Are these and other psychotropic drugs popular because they are easy and cheap, or are they popular because they work? Do they replace therapy or do they complement therapy?

Sometimes they do replace therapy, and they can be just as effective. A course of Prozac, for example, costs two dollars a day. A non-MD therapist gets paid around fifty dollars an hour, and might see a patient four times a month. So medication can be cheaper than therapy, and an HMO may push for this cheaper option. That shouldn't make a difference to you, however. You should be concerned with what works.

Of course, "what works" in this case means what keeps you from getting worse. Since we are talking about acute episodes and not long-term conditions, a short course on medication coupled with three or four visits to a therapist will usually accomplish the HMO's short-term goals.

Before you shy away from medication, do your research. The antidepressants that have come out in the last ten years have been the subject of intense scrutiny, and many of them seem to be living up to their promises. This means that we have to rethink our beliefs about treating emotional disorders like depression. It may be the case that your depression has more to do with a chemical imbalance than your toilet training. If so, it won't do you much good to sit on the therapist's couch for years discussing what's buried deep in your subconscious. Maybe you just need a pill.

The medication vs. therapy debate will go on for years to come, and managed care companies will change their policies toward psychiatric treatment each time one side seems to have the advantage. As a mental health care consumer, you need to be aware of the evolving standards of treatment. You don't want to be caught in the middle, blown from side to side as your HMO's policies change. In partnership with your doctor, find out what works for you. Be prepared to insist on the treatment that works, and be prepared to argue your case if necessary.

What Is a "Carved-Out" Mental Health Program?

Managed care companies were pressured into covering mental health services by employers. Most plans never wanted to deal with this area—that's why most of them have signed contracts with companies that specialize in mental health, agreeing to send all patients who have psychiatric problems to them, rather than treat those problems in-house. This practice is known as "carving out."

Carve-out arrangements make a lot of sense from a business perspective. Many of the HMO's customers will seek mental health services, but nowhere near a majority. Keeping a full staff of therapists, psychiatrists, and licensed social workers on salary to handle what amounts to a sporadic flow of cases would mean wasted time and wasted money. But a mental health group can contract with several managed care plans, ensuring that its waiting rooms are always full.

Carving mental health services out of the health plan also has a few benefits for patients. One of the ways mental health groups sell their services to HMOs is by agreeing to see patients who refer themselves. So if a patient is on the brink of suicide, he can call the mental health group directly.

A patient doesn't have to get a referral from his primary care physician, and then wait for an appointment with a psychiatrist. The mental health group will see him right away, and in most cases provide him with several therapy sessions and a prescription for Prozac. If his suicidal tendencies are mild and related to a specific problem, this treatment will probably be all he needs. If, however, he presents a more serious danger to himself or others, he may be admitted to a hospital.

Direct access to mental health services is a good thing. The ability of primary care doctors to spot and treat mental health problems has been studied repeatedly. They rarely get high marks; either they frequently miss a diagnosis that would be obvious to a specialist, or they make the proper diagnosis, but prescribe an inappropriate treatment. It's not because they didn't pay attention in medical school. In the past, most patients referred themselves to psychiatrists, so the frontline doctors rarely had to spot these conditions.

Now that's changing. Managed care has forced the gatekeeping doctors to bone up on psychiatric conditions, even if mental health has been carved out. Mental health groups frequently offer training to the HMO's primary care doctors on how to spot a patient who needs their services. This means that acute problems will be noticed earlier and treated before they become full-blown crises. The result: fewer patients suffer and the medical group saves money.

Carve-out arrangements can also offer flexible contracts that can save lives. An HMO that doesn't offer mental health services will frequently come across cases that cry out for psychiatric treatment. An anorexic patient, for example, tends to have a number of associated physical health problems that can quickly run up a large bill.

Once such a patient has been admitted to the intensive care unit a couple of times, a cost-conscious HMO will start to look for ways to keep her from overutilizing their services. Even if she doesn't have mental health coverage, the HMO will save money by sending her to a mental health group. The mental health group wants the business, so it is willing to draw up a contract for treating a single patient. The patient gets appropriate treatment, and the HMO can stop fighting a psychiatric problem with physical treatments.

What Should I Watch Out For?

That's the good news about carved-out mental health services. Now for the bad news. Mental health groups that take HMO patients are still managed care. They are paid a flat rate per patient per month, just like the HMO is capitated for covering physical health. You will find the same problems in a mental health group that you will find in your HMO—problems such as caps on visits or denied drugs. In addition, you may encounter even more complex obstacles to getting the care you need. The root of the problems, and your answer to the problems, can be found in the definition of medical necessity. It's harder to prove medical necessity for psychiatric conditions, but when you do, you will hold the key to all the mental health services you need.

Bureaucracy

As you know, your HMO is a bureaucratic institution. The pencil pushers and bean counters seem to call the shots. When mental health is carved out of an HMO, yet another layer of bureaucracy is added. Since the mental health group manages its own financing and administration, you may have to use one set of rules when you deal with the HMO and another when you deal with the mental health group. You may see two sets of rules for referrals, and two sets of rules for appeals.

But even if the HMO and the medical group have an amazing synergy, splitting mental health from physical health creates all sorts of problems. A doctor friend of ours witnessed one of these and told us about it.

"I got called in to see this woman in the ER," he told us. "She's middle-aged and has trouble speaking. Her makeup is applied in this very bizarre way. She can't keep her thoughts on track. It becomes obvious really quickly that she's almost completely out of her mind. Then I find out she's on twenty-six different medications. Twenty-four of them have major central nervous system effects.

"I couldn't find any apparent physical problems, and it didn't take long before I guessed that this woman is delirious from all the medications she's been taking. But her behavior is so erratic that she needs to be in a psychiatric hospital. I couldn't even figure out from her chart why she was on so many meds. Was her delirium caused by the drugs or was it something else? My money was on the drugs. But there was no way to tell except to get her into the hospital and get her off the drugs.

"So I called the mental health carve-out company, and I can't even get a doctor on the phone. It's obvious I'm talking to someone who's going through a checklist to see if there are criteria for admission. She asks me what medications the patient is on, and asks for my assessment. Then an answer comes back in about two hours.

"They didn't want to let her in. I couldn't believe it, but they said that since her problem was caused by the medications (and that was my own assessment), it was a medical problem, and not their problem. That to me is just hairsplitting. She needed a structured environment, not like what we have here. Our patients can walk away at any time. This woman needed to be contained until the drugs cleared her system.

"The president of the carve-out is a personal friend of mine, so I called him directly. He tells me that if he had known it was me he would have approved it right away. I told him that wasn't good enough. Why should my patients be treated any differently? Why isn't there a system in place to deal with this sort of thing?"

Last we heard, the patient was doing well mentally and physically, but was about to enter a bureaucratic minefield. The delirium was indeed caused by the HMO's overuse of medications, so the carve-out group refused to pay. The HMO called it a psychiatric condition, based on the symptoms, and also refused to pay. The patient got letters from both sides saying that she wasn't covered for the hospitalization. As our doctor friend told us, "All sorts of crazy things are about to happen" to this patient.

Everybody in medicine knows that the body and mind are inseparable, but we've allowed the bureaucrats and bean counters to draw this artificial and constantly shifting line between the two. As medical researchers further establish the body-mind connection, managed care policies are taking us back to the nineteenth century.

The patient in the story we just described could have only prepared for this by getting a good advocate. But you can fight this sort of absurd hairsplitting by being active and informed. Here are a few ways to keep mental health bureaucracy from driving you crazy:

- Get your carve-out company's rules and regulations in advance. Find out what their criteria are for seeing you, for treating you, and for appeals. Get this information directly from the carve-out, not from your HMO.

- Keep all your doctors up to date. If you are seeing your PCP for a seemingly unrelated problem, let him know that you are also getting mental health services from the carve-out company. Be especially sure to mention any medications they've given you. You can never assume that one hand knows what the other is doing.

- Be aware of the body-mind connection. If you are getting treatment for both, ask how one treatment may affect the other. Stay clear on how physical treatments can improve or worsen your mental well-being, and vice versa.

- Keep your doctor and therapist on your side. Even if the bureaucrats think they can separate your physical problems from your mental issues, your doctor and therapist know better. If they are your allies, they will do the explaining for you.

Limits on Therapy Visits

When you entered your HMO, you probably took note of how many visits you can make to your doctor. In most health plans, visits to your PCP for specific complaints are not limited. Visits for physical examinations and screening tests are limited, but the number you are allowed is usually reasonable. You probably took this information in, but unless you were already in therapy, you probably didn't take note of the limits, or "caps," on your mental health visits.

In most managed care companies, you get no more than twenty visits a year. At least that's what they tell you in the brochure. In reality, your number of visits to a therapist is determined when you are diagnosed. Unless your case is serious, the best you can hope for is three or four visits to a therapist. If your HMO is generous, you might get as many as six.

Most people will get through their crises in six visits or less. Even before managed care, the average patient only needed six sessions before he felt well enough to discontinue therapy. One psychiatrist who published his own, small-scale survey noticed that many of his patients only came in for a single visit and never returned. When he called those patients, he found that two-thirds of them were doing fine. Simply asking for help had crystallized their problems, given them perspective, and allowed them to heal themselves.

But there are still large cracks in the system that patients can fall through. If a patient suffers three crises a year and gets six visits per crisis, he's close to running out of visits. If he suffers four or more crises per year, that should tell his doctors there is an underlying problem that needs attention. He would be better served by a six-month course of therapy and medication. The HMO would save money by treating his general condition, rather than just managing his crises. It's infuriating, but they just don't do this.

It's amazing how shortsighted managed care can be in cases like this. If a bright young psychiatrist looks at a case and tells the medical director, "Hey, this guy has been in every month this year. I've seen him, and I know I can decrease the crises with a more intensive therapy," you would think that the health plan would jump at the chance. Sadly, that rarely happens.

The case can get tied down by bureaucracy, the accountants might decide it's not in the budget, or the UR doctor might decide that the treatment isn't medically necessary, since the patient isn't getting worse. If a patient like this *does* get worse, he often loses his job, and with it his coverage. Then the health plan doesn't have to treat the patient at all.

The situation is much, much worse for the seriously mentally ill. The system was set up by employers and insurance companies, and since those with severe psychiatric conditions don't usually have jobs, they weren't taken into account when the restrictions on visits were put in place. If a patient with schizophrenia is in a managed care system, he's usually on a parent's or spouse's plan. That means he has an advocate, but that advocate is his only hope.

Even a stable patient with schizophrenia needs twelve visits a year just to check on his medication, leaving only eight visits for therapy. That's nowhere near enough, even for a stable schizophrenic patient. After the severely impaired patient runs out of visits, they usually get transitioned into community mental health services, where they may or may not get adequate treatment. And these are people with insurance! Their families are shocked when they find that their coverage has run out, and there are few avenues for appeal.

Because caps on visits are a benefits issue, and not a medical issue, you won't get far appealing based on medical necessity. But there's a managed care secret that you can use: "flexed benefits." When a managed care company actually wants to bend the rules itself (and this rarely happens) they will take benefit from one place and use it in another. This is called "flexing" the benefit. In a mental health scenario, the simplest way to do this is to shift a benefit you don't think you will need, like inpatient mental health care, to a benefit you do need, like continued therapy visits.

Let's say that you run out of visits at a time when both you and your therapist think that you are close to a breakthrough. Just four more sessions will probably get you there. You've used all your outpatient visits, but you haven't touched your inpatient, or hospitalization, visits. You and your therapist both agree that you probably won't need them. A lot of thought must go into this decision. You don't want to raid your hospitalization reserve unless you can be certain that your case won't require hospitalization.

So you make an offer to your HMO. You declare that you want to flex your inpatient days into outpatient therapy. You have six days of psychiatric hospital stays guaranteed to you. You'd like to flex two of those days into four outpatient visits. That represents a huge savings for the HMO.

Be sure to use this terminology: you want to *flex your benefit*. The plan administrators know exactly what you mean. They'll realize they are dealing with someone who knows the game. If you want to really drive your point home, you could say that if you don't get continued therapy, you will probably need hospitalization. Any HMO would prefer outpatient treatment to hospitalization. You've made their decision very easy and economical for them.

The limits HMOs place on visits display a very archaic attitude toward mental health. Any mental health problem, from mild depression to schizophrenia, should be treated as a medical problem. Arbitrary caps on visits and routine denials of proven drugs are seldom accepted on the medical side, and they shouldn't be accepted on the mental health side.

Don't feel helpless if you have a cap on your visits. There are several things you can do to get the best mental health care from your HMO.

- Create goals for your therapy. Make lists of items you want to cover in your sessions, and make sure you get through those items. Set general goals as well. Share these with your therapist and develop a strategy for getting there.

- Keep track of your visits. If you feel you have accomplished your goals before you complete your course, discuss with your therapist whether you should finish the course or keep the additional visits in reserve. If you are on a medication, remember that your medication visits count just as much as your therapy visits.

- Switch therapists immediately if you aren't getting help. When you only have twenty visits a year, you can't waste any time. Patiently waiting for a breakthrough may have worked in fee-for-service, but in managed care, a therapist has to help you get rapid results.
- Keep a good therapist on your side. If a battle erupts, you will need her help. Don't let this valuable ally slip away.

Denied Drugs

This is going to be an area to watch. Medicines that treat the mind are very expensive, and HMOs are reluctant to keep them in their formularies. In April 1999, one large California managed care company tried to drop Prozac from its list, while another tried to deny its patients access to Zoloft. Both were quickly ordered by the California Department of Corporations, which oversees the health care business in that state, to continue to provide these popular and effective drugs.

This is just one glimpse into the ongoing battle over prescription drugs. It goes far beyond psychiatric medications, but since these drugs are so widely used and so expensive, managed care companies are making a strong effort to limit their use. Prozac has a recommended course of six to nine months. Patients with serious problems should stay on the medication indefinitely. That's not going to happen in managed care unless someone proves that it's medically necessary.

Most Prozac prescriptions in managed care run sixty days. As we've said above, that might be enough to get a patient through a crisis, but it falls short if the patient has chronic emotional problems. And further, the HMO will always try an outpatient treatment first when faced with severely impaired psychotic patients. These treatments *can* work if they use the latest generation of antipsychotic medications in a strictly monitored program. That's good for the patient—psychiatric hospitals are not the best places to live. But if the HMO tries to cut corners further by limiting the drugs or not closely monitoring the situation, serious problems can develop.

It's not just the serious problems, however, that require close monitoring of medication. A huge study of attention deficit disorder, for example, looked at three groups of children who were given three types of treatment: aggressive medication management, aggressive medication management with intensive psychosocial support, and standard community care. The kids on medication did best—and the psychosocial support made little difference.

That's good news for an HMO. They don't need to pay for intensive therapy, just the drugs. But many HMOs will leave the "aggressive management" out of the suggested "aggressive medication management," and just give the kid medication. That won't work. The situation has to be monitored. If the medication is ineffective in a given case, the treatment could make matters worse.

If your HMO drops the ball on medication management, only you can pick it up. If your plan denies a drug that will help, only you can get it approved. Here are some tips for getting and keeping the medication you need.

- Research, research, research. Get help from you therapist, doctor, and pharmacist. Get information from the drug company, and from medical journals. Know your drug and how it affects you.

- Insist on management of your prescription. Your treatment may consist only of medication, with no therapy. If so, you still must see a psychiatrist to check on the progress of your treatment. Don't let your plan send you to a nurse practitioner or primary care doctor for this unless you are perfectly stable. You need the specialized knowledge of a psychiatrist if you have a complicated psychiatric disorder or are starting medications for the first time.

- Set specific goals for your treatment. Write them in your journal. These can be small goals, such as "I want to feel better when I wake up," and large goals, such as "I want to be more assertive and confident at work."

- Monitor your own condition. Keep a journal of your treatment. Take note of how the drug makes you feel, and whether you feel better or worse after you take it.

- Share your findings and goals with your psychiatrist. Discuss openly whether the treatment should continue or be altered.

- Keep all the players on your medical team informed. Be sure your PCP, nurse practitioner, and all specialists you see know that you are on medication. Don't let any stigma you may feel about being treated stand in your way. The medical professionals you deal with won't judge you for being on psychiatric medication.

Substance Abuse Programs

If general mental health services are the stepchild of managed care, substance abuse is the orphan. The HMOs don't want to deal with it, even though it's clear that treating substance abuse will prevent medical problems. Many of the mental health carve-out companies don't want to deal with it, even though it's clear that substance abuse is a psychiatric condition. The issue is that no one has found the magic bullet for dealing with this serious problem. Relapse rates are high, and that means treating the problem can be very risky for capitated companies.

So a third company, separate from the HMO and separate from the mental health carve-out company, usually gets this hot potato of health care. These are tiny companies, when compared to the larger medical groups and mammoth health plans that contract with them, and they specialize in one thing—treating addiction and alcoholism. They aren't very well regulated or closely watched, but in some ways they have proven to be better than what we once had.

The standard of care for substance abuse used to be inpatient care. If you were wealthy, you checked into a treatment clinic out in the country, with rolling hills, lakes, and a golf course. If you were poor, you took what you could get, usually at some place that looked more like a prison than a hospital. If you were a teenager, you might get forced into one of these inpatient settings for months or even years. Companies that provide inpatient drug and alcohol treatment programs made a financial killing, even as research was finding that their effectiveness was questionable.

Inpatient care may succeed in getting patients to dry out, but the ultimate results of locking up the chemically dependent are questionable at best. Studies haven't found a difference between the success of inpatient care and intensive outpatient care. Since outpatient care is cheaper, this is the path your HMO will most likely put you on.

But what works is *intensive* outpatient care. An HMO may review a study that shows how thirty days of intensive outpatient treatment delivers the same results as thirty days of lockup. "Great," they say, "we'll go with the cheaper outpatient treatment." What happens to the intensive part? It gets cut out as the HMO develops a plan, and the savings eventually line someone's pocket.

This puts you back in the position of managing your own treatment team. If you can't take on this role yourself, choose a team captain from among your family and friends. Chemical dependency requires multifaceted treatment. You should get both group and individual therapy. You may find prescription drugs are useful. And any HMO will want you to join a twelve-step program (after all, they're free). If you or your advocate can manage these different aspects of your treatment, you can get the level of intensity needed to resolve your addiction once and for all. But, sadly, you can't expect your HMO to do it all for you.

Here are some general tips to help you through a substance abuse treatment:

- Keep everyone informed. This includes your primary care doctor. You may be nervous about telling her, but she won't judge. She will only show concern and offer help. Don't expect her to ask on her own. Very few doctors, we are sorry to say, do good alcohol and illegal drug histories.

- Investigate your substance abuse carve-out company. Call them directly. Don't assume that your HMO will be able to answer questions about the company it has contracted with. Find out what the mental health group has to offer. Try to take advantage of as many programs as you can.

- Go outside the HMO for help. Find support groups, twelve-step programs, and nonprofit organizations. There are countless free or cheap helping hands for people in recovery.

- Don't give up if you relapse, and don't let your HMO give up on you. Get back into treatment, and be ready to appeal if you have to. During appeals of substance abuse treatment, it's particularly important to have a good advocate.

How Can I Use HEAD for Psychiatric Conditions?

When a psychiatrist asks a patient what's wrong, she is usually prepared for the flood that is sure to follow: "I can't sleep at night. My boss yelled at me. My children hate me. My mother keeps trying to control my life." And so on. In the old days, doctors didn't object to these unorganized lists of complaints. They could expect many of their patients to spend years in therapy, meaning plenty of time to sort out everything out.

Managed care means your time is up. If you have a cap on your visits, you will never see your main problem addressed if you dance around it, listing instead all the little things that bother you. We don't think this is necessarily a good thing—sometimes a patient really does need a platform for their life's grievances. But when the clock is ticking, you have to decide what is most important to you.

This way of approaching therapy is so different from the traditional way that it requires a huge shift in thinking, both for the patient and the therapist. However, you already have the tool you need to accelerate your therapy and bring your therapist along with you. Bring HEAD to your therapy visits, just like you bring it to a visit with your primary care doctor.

It's incredibly easy to adapt HEAD for psychiatric problems. Your therapist, whether he's an MD or not, has been trained to take your history for depression in the same format that your primary care doctor takes a history for a headache. When your therapist sees you are using HEAD, he will know that you are serious about getting help for a specific problem. He will know that you are ready to work with him in a mutual relationship. And he will know you are a patient who won't let the HMO's time limits get in the way of great treatment.

The Psychiatric History

When you use HEAD for your mental health visit, keep two very important topics in mind: your chief complaint and your history of the present illness. In the example above, the patient responds to the therapist's question "What seems to be bothering you?" with a long list of grievances. If you use HEAD, you can still cover everything that's bothering you, but you will be able to do it in a way that lets the therapist move quickly to the root of the problem.

Instead of giving the particulars of your life from the beginning, try to see if you can state the problem in general terms. Instead of saying, "I can't sleep at night. My boss yelled at me. My children hate me. My mother keeps trying to control my life," think about how all these factors create a general mood. What is that mood or feeling? Tension? Panic? Worthlessness? Depression?

A patient using HEAD will give his chief complaint as concisely as possible, and only after the identifying data is out of the way. For example, the patient above might say "I'm a twenty-four-year-old, single website developer. I'm here because of constant tension and stress."

Pause here. You've given your chief complaint. If you also aren't sleeping well at night, if you're having a few problems at work, save those issues for later. The big problem is tension and stress. Too many patients only talk about what happens to them, not about how they feel. In a time-compressed managed care visit, a therapist might not ask the most important question: "How does that make you feel?" They might assume you are depressed when you're actually anxious. This could lead to a misguided treatment.

An opportunity for talking about those other problems is right around the corner. When you get to the history of the present illness, you will have a chance to explain further. As you will remember from chapter 3, the history of the present illness has seven parts: location, quality, quantity or severity, timing, setting, factors, and associated symptoms. They describe the what, where, when, and how of the illness.

For a psychiatric condition, you will need to slightly revise this approach. For example, a complaint like stress has no location. So skip that part for now. Move on to quality. How does the stress feel? Does it make you feel hopeless? Jittery? Uptight? Try to give the doctor the best description of your subjective feeling before you move on to the more objective measurement of quantity or severity.

With quantity or severity, the trick is to try to put a figure on your feelings. The easiest way to do this is to tell the therapist how often you feel a certain way. This is different from "timing," where you explain when the feeling comes and goes. For now, you want to explain how often and how intensely you experience the feeling. For example, you might say, "I have this feeling most of the day on most days." Or you might say, "I have this feeling every few days for a couple of hours a day."

Another way to get at quantity is to compare it to other times you have had this feeling. For example, you might say, "This stress isn't as bad as when I was divorced, but it's worse than when I got fired." A comparison helps the therapist understand what you are going through.

Next, you are on to timing. Does the feeling come up in the morning, evening, or during the day? Does it coincide with other regular events like mealtimes, bedtime, weekends, holidays, or menstruation? If you have noticed a pattern, share this with your therapist. Then you can lead him easily to the next part, setting.

Where are you and what are you doing when this feeling comes up? Who else is there with you? Are there fumes, bright lights, or any other possible physical causes of your feeling? By discussing the setting, you are preparing the therapist to think about a cause of your symptom, and getting ready for the next step, a discussion of the associated factors.

Here is where you can help the doctor decide on a course of action. What people, places, activities, or things do you *know* affect your feeling? What makes it better, what makes it worse, and what makes it change in quality? Just as with a physical symptom, think about particular foods, exercise, and drugs that make the feeling change. If the above patient feels more stress when his mother tries to control his life, he would say that here.

Then you will want to cover associated symptoms. A psychiatric condition can have many associated physical symptoms, such as back pain, headache, and digestive problems. It can also have many associated psychological conditions, such as trouble concentrating or trouble sleeping. Even lack of emotional reactions can be an associated symptom.

As you go through your associated symptoms, do as you would do for a physical symptom. Let the doctor know it's there, then ask if he wants to know more. "I also have severe headaches," you might say. "Do you need more information on that?" If you have proven that you can move quickly through the seven parts of the symptom, he should have no problem letting you continue. If however, he knows you are pressed for time, he may ask you to gloss over the associated symptoms.

The rest of the psychiatric history is very much the same as for the physical history. There will be more questions about your family and about your daily routine, but you already know the basics from chapter 3. The exam will also be different. You will get a series of questions to check your memory and cognitive skills. Don't be frustrated if you can't give a correct answer. Tell the doctor that you don't know or can't remember, then let him know how that concerns you.

Building a Mental Health Team

Once the exam is complete, a psychiatrist, psychologist, or master's level therapist will use the same method to make an assessment as he would for a physical condition. Once the assessment is complete, you and your doctor should be ready to make a decision about your treatment.

Keep in mind everything you have learned about managed mental health care from this chapter. The treatment plan will be for a specific problem, and will lead to a specific goal. The treatment may include drugs, therapy, or both. Be sure to do all the same things you would do if you had a physical condition. Research your problem, find experts, and see an out-of-network specialist for an information-only consultation.

When you have all your information together, look again at your treatment plan. How does it stack up against prevailing medical opinion? Where does it fall short? Who should be on your mental health team?

The specific members of your mental health team will vary depending on who you are and what sort of condition you have, but here's a brief list of the sort of people you want to recruit:

- Your primary care doctor—He's not a mental health specialist, but as coordinator of your care, he should always know what's going on.

- Your therapist—Your therapist will usually not be a doctor. This is one way HMOs try to cut corners. But short of monitoring medication, these non-MD specialists will often do as good a job for mild to moderate cases. They can be nurse practitioners, master's level therapists, licensed social workers, physician assistants, or psychologists. They should also be kept up-to-date about changes in your prescriptions and even about changes in your physical health.

- Your psychiatrist—This specialist normally won't be giving you your therapy sessions. She's there to oversee your case and monitor your medication. Let her know of any changes in your therapy, and of any problems with your medication. There's a good chance this specialist will be rushed. Use HEAD, have your questions ready beforehand, and try to get her interested in your case.

- Your therapy group—Many HMOs will send you to group therapy. Even if the members of your group are annoying, try to make them useful. See what you can learn from them about your case. Find out about their experiences with medication and how they've navigated your HMO's mental health program.

The most important part of leading a mental health team is keeping your physical and mental health tied together. The practice of carving out mental health has the effect of separating mind and body, when they should never be separate. When your physical health players work for one company and your mental health players work for another, however, that's the sort of care you will get. They won't talk to each other, so it falls to you to keep them informed of what's going on outside their specialties.

RESOURCES FOR MANAGED MENTAL HEALTH CARE

American Psychiatric Association
1400 K Street NW
Washington, DC 20005
(202) 682–6000
www.psych.org
A trade association that represents psychiatrists, most of whom are finding that managed care has transformed their practices.

American Psychological Association
750 1st Street NE
Washington, DC 20002
(202) 336–5500
www.apa.org
See website for studies on managed care and mental health.

National Alliance for the Mentally Ill
200 North Glebe Road
Arlington, VA 22203
(703) 524–7600
www.nami.org
The premier advocacy group for the mentally ill. Publishes reports on several large companies that handle mental health treatments.

National Coalition of Mental Health Professionals & Consumers, Inc.
Box 438
Commack, NY 11725
(516) 424–5232
www.nomanagedcare.org
As you may gather from the website address, this group isn't a fan of managed mental health care.

How Will My Teenager's Mental Health Be Treated?

Managed psychiatric care, as we have said, is essentially crisis intervention. It wasn't built for long-term care of chronic problems. But as we all know, adolescence can be one long crisis. Add even a mild depression to that already trying time, and you may have a teenager who needs professional help.

This can happen to anyone, and it doesn't mean the teen has bad parents. One out of five youths age nine to seventeen have a diagnosable emotional or behavioral disorder. Five to 9 percent have extreme functional impairment due to a psychiatric disorder. They are twice as likely as adults to be hospitalized for mental health reasons. When we look at these figures, we see children who need help. When HMOs look at these figures, they see expensive patients.

When HMOs look further, they see the extensive social services system established over the last twenty years. They see a number of state and local programs—school-based counseling, juvenile justice, family counseling services—that were set up to make sure kids didn't fall through the cracks. This gives them an easy way out. They can always shift the burden of care to one of these groups.

Before managed care, too many adolescents were sent to hospitals. Now, you can't get hospitalization until a child becomes a physical threat to himself or others. Of course, by that time he might be in the juvenile justice system, and the HMO still doesn't have to provide care. The child who is abusing drugs will get on a treatment program right away. The child who attempts suicide will get immediate hospitalization. But the child who is flunking out of school is, in the HMO's eyes, the school's problem. The compulsively shoplifting teen is the court's problem. The teen who won't obey his parents is family services' problem.

What the HMOs are looking for are comprehensive "wrap around" services for teenagers, where several agencies pitch in to do a part. Of course, the managed care company really doesn't have to do anything except hospitalize a child who's turned dangerous. This strategy leaves large areas uncovered. Too many moderate cases are allowed to go untreated until they become serious. And then they aren't even treated that well.

If you are a parent with a teen who is experiencing a mental health problem, you can do him a great service by phrasing his problems in medical terms. We aren't saying you have to look up the exact diagnosis, but we are recommending that you think hard about what is causing his behavioral or emotional difficulty.

Dr. Feinberg remembers a patient who would have gotten lost in the system if his mother hadn't stepped up to the plate. The teenager was experiencing more problems than average for his age, but he wasn't on drugs, and he wasn't in a gang. He just refused to go to school. In much the same way that this patient refused to go to school, the managed care company refused to provide the structured environment of a care center where he could get the attention he needed.

Outpatient services don't work for a case like this. If the teenager isn't going to school, why would he go to counseling? The mother tried a number of other avenues in the public sector to get appropriate treatment for her son, and failed at each one. At every setback, she kept Dr. Feinberg informed of the child's worsening condition.

Finally, rather than telling the HMO that the problem was truancy, Dr. Feinberg and the teenager's mother told the HMO that the problem was medical in nature. The teen was missing developmental milestones. His aggressive behavior was on the rise. They painted a picture of a child who was a danger to himself and others. It wasn't easy for the mother to do; most parents would deny to the bitter end that their child is capable of hurting anyone. But this parent was able to put aside her instincts long enough to get her child the care he needed. With a doctor on her side, she was able to get the appropriate treatment.

It can be hard to see your child's problems in terms of medical necessity. So often we hope that these problems are just part of a developmental phase. But you owe it to yourself and your teenager to closely watch the situation and ask the tough questions. When you begin to come up with unpleasant answers, it's time to get your HMO involved. Here are some general tips for guiding your teenager through the wilds of managed mental health care:

- Keep track of the situation. A record of dates and exactly what was said during conversations can help. If the situation is getting worse, you can base your appeal on medical necessity.

- Use public services, but don't let your HMO off the hook. If the administrators at your health plan try to tell you it's not their problem, seek the help they suggest. But if that doesn't work, keep coming back to the HMO with continued demands for help.

- Give your teen private time with your doctor. There may be things he will tell your doctor that he won't tell you. Of course, you want to know as much as possible, but put that aside for a moment. What's important for your child's health is that he get treatment. Sometimes that treatment will go beyond what parents can provide. Sometimes parents have to excuse themselves before treatment can start.

- Pay close attention to warning signs. Drugs, violent behavior, and self-destructive behavior raise red flags at the HMO. Any hint of these warning signs can turn an HMO's "no" into a "yes" very quickly.

- Be an advocate at the HMO, and a parent at home. When you approach your health plan's doctors or reviewers with a problem, don't let them see you as an overreacting parent. Let them know that you aren't just looking for a specific treatment, but that you want what's best for the child. Don't use the doctor or review process to vent about how frustrated you are as a parent.

- Once again, get a doctor on your side. Make him share your concern. Get him to help you with your administrative struggles.

Will My HMO Keep My Therapy Secrets?

As far as ethics and the law goes, nothing has changed in the area of confidentiality between a patient and a therapist. But as a practical matter, the picture looks very different, and this has many patients in therapy very concerned.

When we used therapy in fee-for-service care, we could rest assured that our records would never leave our doctor's office. In many cases, no one even knew that we were going to therapy. No one had to know if we were on medication. Confidentiality was taken for granted, and had a therapeutic effect on patients. No one would know their secrets, and so they felt free to discuss things openly.

But group health insurance relies on open information exchange. While your detailed secrets aren't entered into a computer, your diagnostic codes are. There is also a record of who you saw and what you were prescribed. Even if this is kept from the medical side of the HMO, lab results are open. If you have a lithium level in your blood test, that means you are being treated for a psychiatric disorder.

We talked to one woman who pursued a claim that her large HMO misbilled her. She demanded and received a copy of her records, and was shocked to find her name on a list with forty other patients she didn't know. The list included their names, dates of service, their diagnostic codes, and who they saw. When we looked at this list, we could readily interpret from the codes all sorts of psychiatric conditions attached to the full names of patients.

This is the new reality of your confidential relationship with your therapist. No ethical professional will purposely let this information out. No HMO that doesn't want to face a lawsuit deliberately puts this information in the open. But these are huge systems we're talking about, and the potential for mistakes is always there.

Even in the normal course of doing business, a patient's chart will be handled and reviewed by dozens of doctors, nurses, and file clerks. These employees are required to keep confidentiality, but the fact that unseen eyes are upon our files makes many patients understandably uncomfortable.

And so some patients take their business elsewhere. A recent survey of therapists found that almost 40 percent had at least one patient who paid out of pocket because they were concerned about confidentiality. But this costs money. Shouldn't confidentiality be part of the bargain when we buy health insurance?

Some patients keep their deepest secrets to themselves. We've listened to a number of therapists in managed care report that patients just aren't as open these days. They say that patients are afraid someone in the organization will find out. Some patients even fear that their employer will find out, even though employers don't have the right to their employees' records.

There are obvious problems with each of these confidentiality strategies. Few patients can afford to pay out of pocket, and since they have insurance, they really shouldn't have to. No patient can get the full benefits of therapy while consciously holding back out of fear of exposure. In fact, no strategy will guarantee that you will enjoy complete confidentiality, but we can recommend one way to at least partially protect your secrets.

Again, it involves having your therapist on your side. Discuss openly your concerns about confidentiality, if you have any, before you enter a sensitive topic. You can specifically request that your therapist not make a detailed record of what you are about to discuss. The therapist can be creative, but still truthful, in your chart. For example, instead of writing "patient is involved in extramarital affairs," the therapist can write, "patient reports intimacy problems." Instead of writing "patient reports a past history of sexual abuse," the therapist can write "patient reports past history of severe trauma." Both revised statements are true and medically accurate, however vague.

If a medical professional reads these phrases in a chart before a psychiatric visit, she will be sure to ask what they mean. So the original therapist has done her job by reporting her findings. The next therapist or doctor will do his job by asking the right questions. The patient has gotten the important information out on the table, but doesn't have to worry about someone who is not directly involved in his case gaining very personal information.

But if you take this tactic to improve confidentiality, you must take a more active role in directing your medical team. Your players won't know the details of what's going on just from reading your chart, so you will have to give them a more complete picture. If you decide to request that the chart of your therapy sessions be vaguely written, take extra care to give a clear history to your primary care physician and psychiatrist.

Confidentiality is a hard issue to address. We have all bought into group health insurance, and it seems like our secrets will never again be as closely guarded as they once were. On the other hand, we are more open as a society than we once were. Few people would judge us if they found out we were in therapy or on medication. Our sessions aren't as closed, but our secrets aren't as big a deal. Every patient should be aware of what has happened to confidentiality, but none of us should settle for less from our therapists because the door is ajar.

What Have I Accomplished?

When you treat mental health issues just like you would treat physical health issues, you have taken the first step toward getting complete care. Mental health services shouldn't be an appendix to your managed care plan, and layers of bureaucracy shouldn't stand between you and your therapist. Sadly, mental health is too often an after-thought, and your therapist is typically isolated from the mainstream of health care by carve-out programs.

Being aware that this is taking place gives you an advantage. You know what you are fighting against. You know that your team will need better coaching and more updates from you, the team leader. If you do your research and work with your doctor to make mutual decisions, you won't have to worry about being overmedicated or denied useful drugs.

Finally, when you treat mental health issues just as you would treat physical health issues, you can adopt the tool used so often to deny patients important psychiatric care. Psychiatric care is a medical necessity. It isn't a luxury item or indulgence. It's impossible to maintain your physical health while ignoring your mental condition. When HMOs realize this, both their patients and their bottom line will thrive.

∾ 11 ∾
What's Next?
Possibilities for Managed Care

QUESTIONS THIS CHAPTER ANSWERS
◆ What are the trends to watch?
◆ What does the government have in store?
◆ How will the free market affect my health care?
◆ What trends in medicine should I watch?
◆ What's ideal for managed care?

Very few of even the brightest medical economists could have predicted what happened to health care in the 1990s. Looking back, it's hard to believe that the change to managed care would be so rapid and apparently so complete. When we consider where we've been, we know that our crystal balls will never give us a clear picture of the future.

Just think about how many factors influence the health care service industry. There's government regulation on the federal and state level. Doctors' groups like the AMA want to have a voice. Employers, the real consumers of managed care, will alternate between protesting cuts in care and demanding lower premiums. Not-for-profits like the National Association of Quality Assurance will further improve their quality yardsticks, giving HMOs even more to think about. New drugs and procedures will be developed. And of course, if the economy goes south at any critical juncture in the evolution of managed care, all bets are off.

As a consequence, we wrote this book with only general principles foremost in mind. The specifics of your plan are changing all the time, but if you stick with what's constant, your health plan will respond. Doctors will always use HEAD. Prevention will always be the most reliable road to health. "Medical necessity" will always guide the delivery of services, no matter how the definition changes. Your own research will always be an essential part of your treatment.

But there's no telling how the particulars will change. We can't predict how pharmaceutical companies will react to assaults by politicians and consumers. We can't be sure where the current premium increases will lead. We would love to tell you what's going to happen to Medicare, but even the best minds from both sides of the congressional aisle can't agree on that.

The best we can do for you in the final chapter of this book is to point out a few general trends for you to watch in the years to come. The next best thing we can do is share our dream of a beautiful future for managed care. It's only a dream, and we know that it may never become a reality. But after spending the last several hundred pages telling you how to steer through the harsh realities of managed care, we think it's important to look at what managed care *could* be.

What Are the Trends to Watch?

Managed health care is an amazing industry. No other business in this country affects more lives, or is more affected by so many outside factors. The trends now guiding and being guided by HMOs are too numerous to list here, but we will do our best to outline the ones that will most affect you.

What Does the Government Have in Mind?

Our elected officials think they have found a political gold mine in managed care regulation. That doesn't seem so strange until you look at recent polls that placed health care reform low on the list of issues important to voters. Across the country, governors and legislators make a great show of how committed they are to getting the HMOs in line. The public listens, but in the end lets issues like jobs and education decide their votes.

That hasn't stopped the lawmakers from launching a boatload of proposed legislation for 2000. It's quite a frenzy, with both parties anxious to pass sweeping legislation before it's time for reelection. Why are they suddenly acting so committed, especially when their efforts seem to go beyond the public's interest in the subject? That's easy. Pursuing health reform makes good copy, it's a good way to get your name in the paper, and it makes you look like a compassionate person.

But what makes for good press can often make for bad law. Every regulation has a direct effect on the HMO's bottom line. Medical plans have suffered high losses in recent years, and insurance trade groups claim that additional regulation will force them to further inflate premiums. That means more Americans will be unable to afford insurance. Legislation intended to save lives could very well have the opposite effect.

Something needs to be done, but carefully. The free market shouldn't make all the decisions, but the government shouldn't recklessly pass legislation without balancing business needs against patient needs. In our current system, the two needs are opposed and at the same time intricately linked.

Here's a quick glance at some of the legislation coming down the line, and what it means to you.

Independent Review

Several states have already passed laws requiring managed care to include an outside review board in the appeals process. The National Committee for Quality Assurance (NCQA) will soon make outside review a requirement for voluntary accreditation. Now, as we write, the House of Representatives is considering proposals that would require all HMOs to make outside review available to all their patients in the event of a denial. This will change the players in your appeals process (companies and doctors that provide independent reviews could become very rich), but it doesn't have a direct impact on your chances of success.

An outside appeals board isn't necessarily more liberal than an HMO. It may have its own conflicts of interest. If the outside appeals board is bound to interpret decisions based on your HMO's definition of medical necessity, it is like a jury that has been ordered by the judge to ignore evidence. And where will the mediator or review board get its money? If it comes from the HMO, then the conflict of interest hasn't been removed at all.

This federal law will make Congress look active and concerned, but it won't add much except additional rules and paperwork. Many HMOs are already voluntarily instituting outside review as a customer relations move. As one CEO of a large HMO explained in a statement, "Outside independent review should give our members peace of mind." That just about sums it up. Outside review will make members feel more comfortable without really changing the quality of care they receive.

Don't let your guard slip just because you have been granted an outside review. Every tip we gave in the appeals section still applies. Only your research and arguments will get you the care you need.

The "Prudent Layperson" Law

If you are a prudent layperson and think you need emergency care, Congress wants to make sure you get it. Anecdotal evidence abounds of patients being denied coverage after they visit an emergency room. The worst sort of story involves someone who avoids a visit to the ER because he was denied coverage before.

Critics of this proposed law say that it's unnecessary. HMOs have to provide medically necessary treatment. What could be more medically necessary than an emergency? It's easy to see how in these situations you could get worse without treatment. Why, then, do we have so many claims for emergency care being denied?

Emergency rooms are bad environments for doing paperwork. If you think your family doctor is rushed, take a look at a typical trauma doctor's day. It's not just possible that he'll get something wrong on a chart—it's inevitable. Besides, the ER isn't set up to deliver exact diagnoses of a patient's condition. The primary goal in an emergency is to make the patient stable, and then send him upstairs for fine adjustments.

But if your HMO receives paperwork that contains a misdiagnosis, especially if the treating hospital is out of the network, the first reaction will be to deny coverage. For example, we know one woman who admitted herself to an ER for a life-threatening allergic reaction to peanuts. She'd been in this situation before, and told the doctors exactly what was wrong and what to do.

She walked away in good condition, not knowing that her claim form was being sent off with the diagnosis "contact dermatitis." A skin rash. Of course her health plan was going to turn her down. No "prudent layperson" would see a rash as an emergency, so this proposed law wouldn't have protected her.

Most medically necessary procedures are denied because of bad paperwork and bad communication. But legislation that sets its sights on clerical error is nowhere near as dramatic as laws that make a show of responding to coldhearted denials of treatment to suffering patients.

The good thing about the prudent layperson law is that patients may feel more empowered when making decisions about visiting ERs and urgent care centers. It may save some lives just through providing this confidence. But patients already have the right to self-admit if their life or health is immediately threatened. This law does little more than enforce what we already have.

Medical Necessity—What Is It and Who Decides?

Now here's a debate that really needs to take place. The definition of medical necessity and the power to define the phrase are the keys to managing care, or denying care, as the case may be.

In California, for example, only a doctor can rule requested care as "not medically necessary." This would seem to be logical, but in many other states, a Stanford research project found, lower-level medical professionals will make initial decisions about a case, and a doctor won't get to see it unless it's appealed. Medical directors, the ones who often have the final say, too frequently make decisions not consistent with their own plan's guidelines.

The AMA wants doctors to make the decisions about medical necessity, while the insurance companies want the power to rest with the HMO. In the end, we will probably see a standardized appeals process, which allows the HMO to voice its economic concerns while the doctors voice their medical concerns.

But little will change unless we can decide on a definition of medical necessity. Right now, plans can write their own contractual definition any way they want. They always make the definition deliberately vague. The government could do us a real favor by locking our leading doctors and leading insurers in a room, not allowing them to leave until they come up with a definition that everyone can understand. Until that happens, all you can do is read your contract and use your best understanding to squeeze the best care you can from your HMO.

What Will the Free Market Do to My HMO?

No matter how much regulation the government applies, health care will still be a business. That means the economy, the stock market, and the HMO's balance sheet will have a direct effect on your health. Right now, the economy looks healthy, but managed care companies are trying to come out of a recent slump.

Premium Hikes

During the early to mid-nineties, managed care companies offered rock-bottom prices to beat out their competitors and secure contracts with large employers. This strategy brought up enrollment and completely altered the way health care is delivered in this country. But then HMOs started to bleed red ink. Plans that were once the darlings of investors saw their share prices fall. One well-liked CEO of a managed care company committed suicide as his corporation teetered on the edge of bankruptcy.

The easiest way out was to start sending premiums back on a steady climb. Depending on where you lived, your employer probably saw premium increases of 5 to 10 percent in 1998. Another strategy, which looks good to investors but terrifying to patients, is the practice of squeezing doctors and hospitals for reimbursement rates. The rate at which network doctors are compensated is reviewed each year. Even if the HMO doesn't cut its doctors' compensation, a failure to keep up with steadily climbing medical inflation gives health care providers serious financial problems. This is passed on to you in the form of substandard care.

Mergers

If an HMO is in serious financial trouble, it may start to look for cost savings through a merger. Or it might put itself on the auction block. When a major HMO is acquired or merged, the changes disrupt the lives of thousands of consumers. Doctors and clinics are dropped from the network, sending patients into unfamiliar territory with new providers. Claims processing becomes centralized, sometimes at a remote and insufficiently staffed location, which means appeals can take even longer. And slowly but surely, your options are narrowed.

The search for more efficient delivery of health care services will mean more mergers in the future. The increase in costs, regulation, and use of accreditation will mean that the smaller plans will have less opportunity to survive. We are not far from the day when health care consumers, even in cities, will have a choice between no more than two or three mammoth managed care companies in their area. If that happens, the experiment of applying free market principles to medicine will be a complete failure.

It's important to monitor how your HMO is performing as a business. Most of the large ones are publicly owned, so you can get everything from their quarterly earnings reports to the CEO's salary. If your plan starts to stumble, its losses will eventually trickle down to you. You want to be informed and prepared should this happen.

What Trends in Medicine Should I Watch?

Call us biased, but we think the trends that promise real improvement in managed care are coming from innovative approaches to medicine rather than from government regulation or business decisions. It's taken doctors and medical directors a long time to adjust to managed care, but they are learning and changing. Their new approaches will be the ones that guide managed care to new levels.

Superspecialized Clinics

The original vision of managed care was the staff model, where everything was under one roof. But as the last ten years have shown us, patients don't generally like staff models, and administrators have a difficult time cramming the entire world of medicine into one building. These models have a few advantages—your medical team is all in one place—but they don't match the reality of modern medicine.

New treatments are usually developed and tested by small teams working in a single location. After they publish their clinical trials, they get to cash in on their innovation. Other doctors will learn the procedure and it will slowly spread. But the best, most practiced, and sometimes cheapest place for this procedure will be with the ones who originated it.

These pioneering doctors are so specialized that an HMO would never think of putting them on the network. Instead, it will offer last year's model to its patients, even if that outdated treatment is invasive, costly, and requires a series of follow-up visits for therapy or management of complications.

But as the superspecialists adapt to the managed care environment, they are becoming more willing to negotiate lower fees with HMOs just to get the business and practice. As patients become more aware of what's happening in medicine, they are demanding the latest proven treatments. If all three parties sit down and hammer out a plan, all three can win.

Shouldice Hospital in Toronto, for example, the subject of a Harvard Business School case study, specializes in surgical treatment of hernias. A hernia can be a chronic, incredibly painful problem that requires years of treatment. But if the patient gets the right operation the first time, along with proper education about how to help healing take place, the problem can be resolved quickly and cheaply.

If you run through the numbers, in some cases it's actually cheaper for an HMO to fly a patient out to the superspecialists at this hospital for an operation and a series of seminars on his condition. If the treatment works, and the success rates of this venture indicate that it probably will, then all the HMO has had to do is write a check. Complications, physical therapy, and follow-up visits are minimized. The HMO saves money, the patient gets the best care, and the hospital gets business.

We hope that our specialist colleagues will go even further in setting up superspecialized clinics and services, and making deals with HMOs to attract patients. The only reason it hasn't happened so far is that we doctors can be great with patients but horrible at business. Managed care is forcing that to change.

The Specialized "Generalist"

Before managed care, no one paid attention to generalists. The family practice doctor was rarely studied, infrequently published, and often looked down on by the medical establishment. Now she's driving the bus.

Under managed care, "generalist" is quickly becoming an outdated term. The primary care physician specializes in outpatient service, common problems, and disease management. This can be great for the practice of medicine as a whole. Someone who is capable of coordinating treatment between specialists, who knows just enough about each specialty to guide a patient through them, is in a unique position. She can see the whole picture, and find new ways specialists can work together.

Throughout this book we have asked you to be the captain of your own medical team. Someday, however, a new breed of primary care physician will emerge, one who specializes in seeing the big picture. Already, medical schools are preparing generalists for this role, with even more emphasis on previously neglected areas like psychiatry and sustained treatment of chronic illness.

This can be very good news for patients. More team members and better coordination usually translates into less invasive procedures. As more information about a particular case filters down to the generalist from the specialists, the generalist will find a wider range of options than any of those specialists would have found on their own. And the front-line generalists are usually much better at forming partnerships with patients.

This trend toward redefining and reemphasizing the primary care doctor isn't just good news for patients. It's great news for the bottom line. Specialists will become less directly involved with patients as PCPs become better at coordinating care. That leaves them free for other referrals, saving the HMO money.

When you bring the team-management techniques you have learned in this book to your visits with your PCP, you are helping push this trend forward. You aren't just helping yourself—you're helping the HMO and your doctor evolve.

Two Modest Proposals for Managing Managed Care

It's time for the truth to be told. We've guided you through all you need to know to make managed care work for you, but we've left something out. The system we describe won't work for everybody all at the same time. That is, if everybody in managed care used the methods we recommend in this book, the entire system would go bankrupt.

Managed care came along because everyone realized that if there wasn't some entity to tell patients "no," health care costs would drive the entire nation to the poorhouse. There's no way around that. We can't give the maximum in health care to each individual. We have to start thinking about the health of the nation. Someone has to make hard choices.

When President Clinton's nationalized health insurance proposal failed, the responsibility for saying "no" went to big business. There's an ethical problem inherent in that, which we are all aware of. When a patient's health suffers because of a denied treatment, someone else profits. You can't remove this conflict of interest from the current system. Even nonprofit HMOs have a hard time avoiding this ethical dilemma.

So who should say "no"? Consumers have said loud and clear that we don't want big government to play this role. But someone has to. We need a system in which treatment policies can be established by those who are close to the people the decisions affect, and who are shielded as much as possible from conflicts of interest.

We believe the hard decisions should fall to our individual communities. Each region, say a county, covered by managed care should take the initiative to appoint a body composed of community leaders, insurance representatives, doctors, employers, AARP representatives, and union leaders. This body should make the hard choices for its own community.

We hate the idea of rationed care. But realistically, there's only so much money to go around. HMOs are already rationing care, but they're doing it with an eye to profits, without thinking about the best interests of the community at large. The rational way to ration care is to prioritize treatments and drugs, with the most important—immunizations, screenings, and insulin, for example—rising to the top tier of the list. There should always be enough money to cover the most important procedures. If there's money left, then procedures and drugs down toward the bottom of the list—circumcisions and heroic resuscitations for terminal patients, for example—can be covered as well. Oregon has been working with a list like this for Medicare and Medicaid patients for years. When it was first introduced, critics howled about how this amounted to rationing care. The response was simple: there's just not enough money to do otherwise.

We don't want big business to assume responsibility for a list like this. We don't want big government telling us who lives and who dies. That's why we think it should fall to responsible leaders who live in the community. No one wants to deny a lung transplant to a dying smoker. But everyone on the sort of board we envision would agree that smoking prevention programs should be higher on the list than lung transplants for smokers. And in the end, we will probably find that prevention will save enough money to let us splurge on lung transplants for those few people left who do smoke.

It looks like rationed care, but it's actually prioritized care. When the list is agreed upon, it is left to the HMOs to work within those community guidelines. The HMO will still take in a lot of money from its premiums. The only difference is that the community gives the HMO minimum guidelines for where the money should go. If the HMO finds ways to save money and still meet those guidelines, great. It can put some toward profit, and some toward providing treatments further down the list.

This scenario leaves plenty of room for competition. Plans will have to work with the same list, but the ones that provide the most efficient care and the best prevention will have money left over to offer procedures further down the list. They can use that as a selling point to employers, individuals, and Medicare patients, who will finally have a direct and simple way to compare one plan to another.

We admit we are dreaming. Hundreds of millions of lobbying dollars are lined up against managed care reform. Even the powerful lobbying forces of the AMA can't compete against that sort of political muscle. We are certain that community-based, prioritized care planning can work if executed thoughtfully. We are also realistic about its chances of ever getting a trial.

The other way doctors and conscientious health plans can manage managed care is immediately available. It's just a matter of common sense. When Dr. Feinberg was a psychiatric resident, he got his first chance to run a children's clinic. He treated more patients, and achieved higher patient satisfaction levels, than any of the other clinics in the local system, most of which had been around for years.

When he was offered the chance to run another clinic, Dr. Feinberg was asked by the administrators what he needed to get the same results. He said he needed apples, graham crackers, and coffee. The idea was to try to give families all they needed in one long afternoon, rather than keep them coming back over several days. The snacks were just there to keep patients from getting hungry during the session.

Dr. Feinberg might have made only small changes at the first clinic he ran, but they had a large impact. He had his employees answer the phones so the patients wouldn't have to wander through voice mail. He redistributed the work among his staff members and set up one-stop sessions for families. Eventually his staffers were able to see and help eight times as many patients as they had before his arrival. The patients were happy, the administrators were happy, and the staff was happy knowing they were getting more done and done well.

All Dr. Feinberg had done was think about what he would have wanted for his own family—efficient, friendly care that gives quick results.

Eventually, managed care will learn about customer service. Real people will answer the phone. Clinics will pop up in places where normal people with jobs can easily stop in for an appointment. Doctors will go to where people work to make sure they are in a healthy environment. The entire industry will relearn the concept of bedside manner.

Until that happens, you will have this guide to make sure cost cutting doesn't interfere with your health. You have a preventive plan that will keep you from becoming a victim. You have the resources, abilities, and skills to get you through a managed care crisis. While everyone from congressmen to physicians wonders and worries about where health care is headed, you can rest assured that you will get the best care no matter where it goes.

~ Appendix A ~
Useful Forms
(All these forms are available at www.drtheo.com)

◆ *History Form*
◆ *History Form for Kids*
◆ *Prescriptions, Over-the-Counter Drugs, and Supplements Form*
◆ *Sleep History Form*
◆ *Release of Medical Information Form*

In chapter 3, we outlined the medical history. We know that it's a lot of information to keep together, so we've provided this form to fill out before you go to the doctor. A lot of your past medical history will be covered by the form you fill out in the waiting room, but these forms often omit important questions. Compare this form to the one you are handed at your doctor's office or clinic and be sure to mention anything that their form misses.

Some doctors will appreciate this written form; others won't see a need to put it in your official records. But either way, this form should never replace the oral history.

HISTORY FORM

IDENTIFYING DATA
See page 52.
Age: _____
Ethnic background: _____
Place of birth: _____
Marital status: _____
Occupation: _____
Religion: _____
Sexual orientation: _____

SOURCE OF REFERRAL
See page 54.
Who sent you? _____

SOURCE OF HISTORY
See page 55.
Any other medical records? _____

_____

CHIEF COMPLAINT
See page 55.
Why did you come in? _____

_____

PRESENT ILLNESS
See page 56.
Location: _____
Quality: _____
Quantity/severity: _____
Timing: _____
Setting: _____
Factors: _____
Associated symptoms: _____

_____

PAST HEALTH

See page 64.

General state of past health: _____

_____

Childhood illnesses: _____

_____

Past adult illnesses: _____

_____

Past psychiatric conditions: _____

_____

Accidents and injuries: _____

_____

Operations and hospitalizations: _____

_____

CURRENT HEALTH

See page 65.

Allergies: _____

_____

Immunizations: _____

_____

Screening tests: _____

Last HIV screening: _____

Exposure to toxins: _____

Exercise: _____

Other activities: _____

Sleep quality: _____

Special diets: _____

Caffeine intake (coffee, tea, or cola per day): _____

Smoking habits (in "pack-years"): _____

Drug intake (prescription, over-the-counter, vitamins and supplements, and illegal drugs. Be sure to bring your supplements and over-the-counter drugs with you. If you can't, use the medications form in this appendix): _____

_____

_____

_____

FAMILY HISTORY

See page 67.

Check any of the following conditions that appear in your family:

Alcoholism: _____

Anemia: _____

Arthritis: _____

Cancer (type): _____

Diabetes: _____

Drug addiction: _____

Epilepsy: _____

Headaches: _____

Heart disease: _____

High blood pressure: _____

Kidney disease: _____

Mental illness: _____

Stroke: _____

Tuberculosis: _____

SOCIAL HISTORY

See page 68.

Who lives with you? _____

_____

Important life moments: _____

_____

_____

Future plans: _____

_____

_____

NOTE: Doctor will probably ask about sexual history, including number of partners, sexual problems, and history of STDs, if any.

REVIEW OF SYSTEMS

See page 68.

List problems not related to your chief complaint by system: _____

_____

_____

_____

Recent weight change? _____

Weakness, fatigue, or fever? _____

Skin, hair, and nails: _____

Head: _____

Eyes: _____

Nose: _____

Mouth and throat: _____

Neck and glands: _____

Breasts: _____

Respiratory: _____

Cardiac: _____

Gastrointestinal: _____

Urinary: _____

Genitals: _____

Peripheral vascular (circulation through legs): _____

Musculoskeletal: _____

Neurologic: _____

Hematologic: _____

Endocrine: _____

Psychiatric: _____

HISTORY FORM FOR KIDS

The adult history works for children as well, but as we discussed in chapter 8, children have special needs, and the doctor may ask some special questions.

If you want your doctor to have a complete history for your child in ten minutes, take some time to fill out both the preceding history form and the one below before your visit.

IDENTIFYING INFORMATION

See page 209.

In addition to identifying information for the adult history, include:

Nickname: _____

Parents' marital status: _____

Parents' names: _____

Was child adopted? Are medical records available? From where? _____

_____

Parents' occupations: _____

_____

_____

CHIEF COMPLAINT

See page 209.

In addition to information for adult history, include:

Source of information (parent, babysitter, teacher): _____

_____

PRESENT ILLNESS

See page 210.

In addition to information for adult history, include:

Family members' reactions to child's illness: _____

_____

PAST HEALTH

Be sure doctor has a record of the following:

Birth history

See page 212.

Prenatal history, including complications or harmful substances taken during pregnancy: _____

Natal history, including difficulty of delivery, birth order, and complications:

Neonatal history, including child's illnesses or feeding and breathing problems: _____

Feeding history

See page 212.

Nursing infants—length and frequency of feedings, supplements, complications: _____

Bottle-fed infants—type, concentration, and amount of formula.
Frequency of feedings: _____

Digestion, infants—report problems like regurgitation, colic, and diarrhea:

Weaning—When and how was child weaned? What were his first solid foods?

General eating habits (for children): _____

GROWTH AND DEVELOPMENTAL HISTORY
See page 213.

Height and weight:

Date	Height	Weight
_____	_____	_____
_____	_____	_____
_____	_____	_____
_____	_____	_____
_____	_____	_____
_____	_____	_____
_____	_____	_____
_____	_____	_____
_____	_____	_____
_____	_____	_____
_____	_____	_____
_____	_____	_____
_____	_____	_____
_____	_____	_____

Developmental milestones:

Held up head while lying down on: _____ (date)

Rolled over from front to back on: _____ (date)

Rolled over from back to front on: _____ (date)

Sat up with support on: _____ (date)

Sat up alone on: _____ (date)

Walked with support on: _____ (date)

Said first word on: _____ (date)

Said combination of words on: _____ (date)

Said first sentence on: _____ (date)

Tied shoes without help on: _____ (date)

Dressed without help on: _____ (date)

Sleep
Use sleep history form (see page 293) with your child whenever possible.

Toilet training

Went to bathroom alone on: _____ (date)

Bedwetting patterns (if any): _____

_____

Terms used with child for defecation and urination: _____

_____

Speech

Signs of stuttering, hesitation, or other problems: _____

Schooling

Grade: _____

Environment: _____

Any social or academic problems? _____

_____

CURRENT HEALTH

See page 215.

Follow current health history for adults, but be sure to inform doctor of the following immunizations:

To age two

Diphtheria, tetanus, pertussis (DTP)	Dates: _____	_____	_____	_____	_____
Polio (IPV or OPV)	Dates: _____	_____	_____	_____	
Measles, mumps, rubella (MMR)	Dates: _____	_____			
Hib (influenza)	Dates: _____	_____	_____	_____	
Hepatitis B (Hep B)	Dates: _____	_____	_____		
Vericella (chicken pox):	Dates: _____				

Age two to thirteen

Diphtheria, tetanus, pertussis (DTP)	Dates: _____	_____	_____	_____	_____
Polio (IPV or OPV)	Dates: _____	_____	_____	_____	
Measles, mumps, rubella (MMR)	Dates: _____	_____			
Vericella (if child has not had chicken pox):	Dates: _____				

PRESCRIPTIONS, OVER-THE-COUNTER DRUGS, AND SUPPLEMENTS FORM

We recommend that you always take all your medications and supplements to the doctor with you, but we realize that this isn't always practical. When you can't, this form is the second best thing. Fill it out each time you go to the doctor's office. Remember to be careful and complete—drug interactions can be deadly!

MEDICATION & SUPPLEMENT LIST

Name _____

Date updated _____

List all of the nonfood items you consume in the form below. For products that have multiple ingredients, be sure to bring in the bottles to your doctor for closer inspection.

Name of medication, supplement, or over-the-counter product.	Date started	Taken how often (e.g., twice daily, four times per week, once per month)	Amount taken each dose (milligrams)

SLEEP HISTORY FORM

The sleep history can be crucial in figuring out an exact diagnosis, but it's one that both doctors and patients have trouble with. Patients are too often vague or can't remember details, and doctors too often don't have the right questions.

This form will help. If you are having general sleep problems, make fourteen photocopies and keep them next to your bed. Each morning when you wake up, fill out the form whether you had trouble sleeping the night before or not. When you go to your doctor's office, bring forms for as many nights as you can. It's best to have at least a week's record.

Sleep record for the evening of (day of week and date): _____

Did you take a nap yesterday? If so, how long did it last? _____

Time of evening you went to bed: _____

Approximate time in bed before you fell asleep: _____

Was falling asleep particularly difficult or easy, or did you fall asleep normally? _____

_____

Did you wake up during the night? How many times? _____

_____

How long, approximately, did you stay awake each time? _____

_____

How difficult was it to go back to sleep (difficult, easy, or normal?): _____

_____

Approximately how much sleep did you get? _____

What time did you wake up in the morning? _____

Do you feel more rested or less rested than normal? _____

Was the quality of sleep you did get better or worse than normal? _____

_____

RELEASE OF MEDICAL INFORMATION FORM

You should keep a copy of your medical records. Besides having the safety of a spare set (these important documents get lost more often than you would think), you can use your set to update new doctors about your history and give copies to everyone on your medical team.

Paperwork moves slowly through HMOs. There's no guarantee that a specialist or new doctor will have received your records by the time your appointment rolls around. Use this form to request a set of your records, and update that set every time you have a significant visit.

Patient's Name: _____

Medical Record Number (if known): _____

Birthdate: _____ / _____ / _____

Please release the above patient records to (check all that apply):

_____ Doctor: _____

Address: _____

_____

phone: _____

_____ Insurance Company Name: _____

Address: _____

_____

phone: _____

_____ Your Name: _____

Address: _____

_____

_____

This patient was treated by your staff from (enter date):

_____ / _____ / _____ until (enter date): _____ / _____ / _____

If you have any questions I can be reached at (phone number)

(_____) _____ – _____

_____   _____ / _____ / _____
Signature of Patient/Parent/ Guardian   date

∽Appendix B∽
Disease Risks by Age Group

Do you have a "retirement plan" for your health? Planning for good health thirty or forty years down the road is where prevention can really pay off. How do you do this? How can you predict where to put your efforts into staying healthy?

Determining your risks by your age group is the first step, and the charts below will help. Once you know what you should be concerned about *right now*, take this information to your doctor, along with your personal medical history, your family medical history, and your current lifestyle habits. With your doctor, develop a plan that will guide your lifestyle changes and your screening schedule. A list of disease-specific interventions appears in appendix C.

Mortality data from National Vital Statistics System. Final 1996 data (most current).

ALL AGES

Rank	Top Ten Causes of Death	Number per year
	All causes	2,314,690
1	Heart diseases	733,361
2	Cancers (all types combined)	539,533
3	Stroke	159,942
4	Chronic obstructive pulmonary (lung) disease	106,027
5	Accidents and adverse effects	94,948
5a	Motor vehicle accidents	43,649
5b	All other accidents and adverse effects	51,299
6	Pneumonia and flu	83,727
7	Diabetes	61,767
8	HIV	31,130
9	Suicide	30,903
10	Chronic liver disease	25,047
	All other causes	448,305

AGES 1–4 YEARS

Rank	Top Ten Causes of Death	Number per year
	All causes	5,948
1	Accidents and adverse effects	2,147
1a	Motor vehicle accidents	820
1b	All other accidents and adverse effects	1,327
2	Congenital (birth) anomalies	638
3	Cancers (all types combined)	424
4	Homicide and legal intervention	420
5	Heart diseases	217
6	Pneumonia and flu	168
7	HIV	147
8	Infections in the blood	83
9	Benign neoplasms, carcinoma in situ, and neoplasms of uncertain behavior and of unspecified nature	70
10	Certain conditions originating in the perinatal period	60
	All other causes	1,574

AGES 5–14

Rank	Top Ten Causes of Death	Number per year
	All causes	8,330
1	Accidents and adverse effects	3,433
1a	Motor vehicle accidents	1,980
1b	All other accidents and adverse effects	1,453
2	Cancers (all types combined)	1,028
3	Homicide and legal intervention	514
4	Congenital anomalies	457
5	Heart diseases	334
6	Suicide	302
7	HIV	177
8	Chronic obstructive pulmonary (lung) disease	165
9	Pneumonia and flu	136
10	Benign neoplasms, carcinoma in situ, and neoplasms of uncertain behavior and of unspecified nature	85
	All other causes	1,699

AGES 15–24

Rank	Top Ten Causes of Death	Number per year
	All causes	32,443
1	Accidents and adverse effects	13,809
1a	Motor vehicle accidents	10,576
1b	All other accidents and adverse effects	3,233
2	Homicide and legal intervention	6,548
3	Suicide	4,358
4	Cancers (all types combined)	1,632
5	Heart diseases	969
6	HIV	413
7	Congenital (birth) anomalies	382
8	Chronic obstructive pulmonary (lung) disease	237
9	Pneumonia and flu	203
10	Stroke	167
	All other causes	3,725

AGES 25–44

Rank	Top Ten Causes of Death	Number per year
	All causes	147,180
1	Accidents and adverse effects	27,092
1a	Motor vehicle accidents	14,482
1b	All other accidents and adverse effects	12,610
2	HIV	21,894
3	Cancers (all types combined)	21,685
4	Heart diseases	16,567
5	Suicide	12,602
6	Homicide and legal intervention	9,322
7	Chronic liver disease	4,210
8	Stroke	3,442
9	Diabetes	2,526
10	Pneumonia and flu	2,029
	All other causes	25,811

AGES 45–64

Rank	Top Ten Causes of Death	Number per year
	All causes	378,054
1	Cancers (all types combined)	131,455
2	Heart diseases	102,369
3	Accidents and adverse effects	16,717
3a	Motor vehicle accidents	7,749
3b	All other accidents and adverse effects	8,968
4	Stroke	15,468
5	Chronic obstructive pulmonary (lung) disease	12,847
6	Diabetes	12,687
7	Chronic liver disease	10,743
8	HIV	8,053
9	Suicide	7,762
10	Pneumonia and flu	5,706
	All other causes	54,247

AGES 65 AND OVER

Rank	Top Ten Causes of Death	Number per year
	All causes	1,713,725
1	Heart diseases	612,199
2	Cancers (all types combined)	382,988
3	Stroke	140,488
4	Chronic obstructive pulmonary (lung) diseases	91,470
5	Pneumonia and flu	74,979
6	Diabetes	46,376
7	Accidents and adverse effects	30,830
7a	Motor vehicle accidents	7,784
7b	All other accidents and adverse effects	23,046
8	Kidney diseases	21,077
9	Alzheimer's disease	20,869
10	Infections in the blood	17,337
	All other causes	275,112

~ Appendix C ~
Condition-Specific
Preventive Interventions

This section provides a concise summary of the latest knowledge concerning prevention of some of the most common serious medical conditions. No matter how far medical science goes in curing these conditions, the best way to avoid the risk they present is through prevention.

The incidence rates of some of these conditions—diabetes, osteoporosis, osteoarthritis—are climbing steadily. At the same time, deaths from injuries and heart attacks are on the decline. All told, chances are that most of us will suffer from one or more of the conditions on the following list at some time in our lives. Think about that if you ever feel like your preventive plan isn't worth your time.

We can't cover prevention for each and every illness, but we will cover preventions for these common conditions in this appendix:

- Heart disease and stroke
- Cancers: The top ten, and interventions for lung, colon, breast, and prostate cancer
- Diabetes
- Osteoarthritis
- Osteoporosis
- Memory loss

How Can I Prevent Heart Disease and Strokes?

There are 1.5 million heart attacks per year and 733,000 deaths from heart attacks in this country. Seven hundred thousand people suffer strokes each year in the United States and 160,000 die from strokes.

Half of all American men and a third of American women under age forty will develop coronary heart disease at some point in their lives.

Although we should all take preventive measures to prevent heart disease and stroke, the following people are at higher risk, and need to take special care:

- Men older than forty-five and women over fifty-five.

- Anyone with high blood pressure. If the upper number (systolic) is above 140, or if the lower number (diastolic) is above 90, then your blood pressure is too high and will damage your arteries. Recent evidence suggests that even blood pressure readings as low as 130/85 can be damaging and may require treatment.

- Smokers, even "occasional" smokers. About half of the cases of heart disease and stroke are linked to smoking.

- Anyone with high LDL ("bad") cholesterol (130 or higher).

- Anyone with low HDL ("good") cholesterol (35 or lower).

- Anyone with diabetes (either insulin dependent or non–insulin dependent).

- Anyone with a first-degree relative (parent, sibling, or child) who has suffered heart disease. This is especially true if a heart attack occurred in a male first-degree relative before he was fifty-five, or if it occurred in a female first-degree relative before she reached sixty-five.

- Anyone who gets less than twenty minutes of aerobic exercise three times per week.

- Anyone who is overweight (especially when the waist-to-hip ratio is greater than 0.95 in men and greater than 0.85 in women). This ratio is easy to calculate. Using a tape measure, find the narrowest region of the waist in inches and divide this number by the measurement of the widest region of the hips and buttocks.

- Anyone who eats a diet high in saturated fat, "trans" fat (see chapter 5), and cholesterol.

- Anyone with a high degree of hostility and anger.

- Anyone who has an elevated level of homocysteine, fibrinogen or C-reactive protein, or Lp(a) (a subtype of cholesterol not detected on a regular cholesterol test). There are special blood tests for these levels that are indicated for people with high cholesterol or who have a family history of heart disease. Most HMOs do not yet cover these tests so you may have to pay for these yourself.

Prevention Strategies

- Don't smoke. If you smoke, all bets are off. There's no safe exposure and you can't negate the effects of smoking by being "good" in all of the other areas. Remember, if you smoke, you have a 100 percent chance that the tobacco is adversely impacting your health and a one in three chance you'll die from a smoking-related disease. Most smokers do not die suddenly but linger with disability for years before their premature death.

- Lose weight. If you are overweight, especially if you have a large waist-to-hip ratio, see the diet and exercise sections of chapter 5.

- Get a complete profile of your blood cholesterol at least once every five years starting at age twenty. Start sooner if there's a strong family history of high cholesterol. If your cholesterol is high, treat it aggressively with lifestyle improvements; if necessary, include medication in your treatment plan. Cholesterol-lowering medicine has proven to be one of the most beneficial and lowest risk treatments in medicine today.

- Get your levels of homocysteine, fibrinogen (or C-reactive protein), and Lp(a) level checked if you have a family history of heart disease or a personal history of high cholesterol. Abnormalities in one or more of these independent risks for artery blockage may require special treatment. For elevated homocysteine, the B vitamins B_{12} and folate, sometimes in high doses, are the main treatment. For elevated fibrinogen, the main treatments are supplemental omega-3 fatty acids and, for women, estrogen. For high Lp(a) levels, aggressive LDL cholesterol lowering is the main treatment; sometimes high-dose niacin (vitamin B_3) is used.

- Get your blood pressure checked at least four to six times each year, at different times of the day, even if you don't have high blood pressure. Have it checked during every doctor's visit. Use the automatic machines you can find in many pharmacies. Don't delay in starting a course of prescription blood pressure medicine if your doctor recommends it. Most modern blood pressure medicines have no significant side effects in most users. The potential results of *not* treating high blood pressure include heart attack, stroke, impotence, dementia, and kidney and eye damage.

- Ask your doctor if taking aspirin is right for you. For some, the risk of internal bleeding from aspirin outweighs the potential benefits.

- Consider supplements including soy isoflavones and the antioxidant group, which includes vitamin A (or mixed carotenoids), mixed vitamin C (in a mixed form like citrus bioflavonoids), mixed vitamin E (also called mixed tocopherols), selenium, pycnogenol, grape seed extract, CoQ-10, alpha lipoic acid, glutathione, green tea extract, and N-acetylcysteine.
- Eat a preventive diet and get plenty of exercise. Read the diet and exercise sections of chapter 5.

How Can I Prevent Cancer?

Cancer causes 540,000 deaths in this country every year. The number of cases continues to climb but the death rates for some cancers have actually improved, thanks to earlier detection and better treatments. People fear cancer more than any other disease, partly because the treatments for cancer (surgery, chemotherapy, and radiation) are invasive and partly because there is often chronic and unremitting pain associated with the later stages of most cancers.

Fortunately, over 50 percent of cancer cases are avoidable. The vast majority of lung cancer cases (the number-one cancer killer) could have been prevented if the patient had quit smoking and stuck with it. Overall, smoking causes about 30 percent of cancer cases, so tobacco is by far the biggest culprit. Excessive alcohol intake and low consumption of fruits and vegetables are also major contributors.

Many cancers aren't killers if they are caught early. Colon cancer is about 95 percent curable if caught in its earliest stage. Pushing cancer from your mind won't make it go away. Only prevention can lower your chances of contracting or dying from this disease.

Ask the average person what health condition they fear most and the usual response is "cancer." What can be done to prevent these cancers? Lots. Did you know that half of these deaths are completely preventable? We hear about general prevention strategies all the time, but the message just doesn't sink in for most people. Here are the risk factors and prevention strategies for the four most lethal cancers.

Lung Cancer Risk Factors

- Cigarette smoking
- Asbestos exposure

- Secondhand smoke
- Increasing age
- Diets low in fruits and vegetables

Lung Cancer Preventive Interventions

- Don't smoke!
- Avoid secondhand smoke.
- If you live or work in an older building, make sure it has been evaluated for loose asbestos fibers.
- Eat a healthy diet and exercise (see diet and exercise sections of chapter 5).
- Boost your immune system with good sleep, prayer, meditation, social and community connectedness (chapter 5).
- Consider the supplements listed in the supplement section of chapter 5.

Colon and Rectal Cancer Risk Factors

- Family history (colon or rectal cancer in a parent, sibling, or child)
- Increasing age, especially after age 50
- History of colon polyps
- European Jewish (Ashkenazi) heritage

The Ten Most Lethal Cancers

Type of Cancer	1998 U.S. Deaths (estimated)
Lung/bronchus	160,000
Colon/rectum	56,500
Breast (about 400 deaths are among males)	44,200
Prostate (male only)	39,200
Pancreas	28,900
Non-Hodgkin's lymphoma	24,900
Leukemias	21,600
Ovary (female only)	14,500
Stomach	13,700
Brain/nervous system	13,300

- Sedentary lifestyle
- Cigarette smoking
- Diets high in saturated fat or red meat
- Diets low in fiber, fruits, vegetables, beans, and whole grains

Colon and Rectal Cancer Preventive Interventions

Starting at age fifty, get a colonoscopy (inspection of the full colon) every five years. Less accurate is a sigmoidoscopy (inspection of the last third of the colon) or a double contrast barium enema every five years. Least accurate is a stool blood test every year, which misses far too many causes of cancer.

- Don't smoke!
- Avoid secondhand smoke.
- Ask your doctor if taking aspirin is right for you. For some, the risk of internal bleeding from the aspirin outweighs the potential benefits.
- Get enough calcium (see the supplements listed in the supplement section of chapter 5).
- Boost your immune system with good sleep, prayer, meditation, social, and community connectedness (chapter 5).
- Eat a healthy diet and exercise (see diet and exercise sections of chapter 5). Lack of exercise appears to be strongly related to colon cancer. Diets higher in fiber, folic acid, and selenium appear protective.

Breast Cancer Risk Factors

- Increasing age
- Family history (breast cancer in a mother, daughter, or sister)
- Benign breast disease (with proliferation, atypical hyperplasia or calcifications)
- Having a first child at thirty or older or having no children
- Early menarche (first menstrual period)—that is, before age twelve
- Late menopause (age fifty or older)
- Alcohol (even one drink a day can significantly increase risk)
- Obesity
- Sedentary lifestyle

Breast Cancer Preventive Interventions

- Get a breast exam by a health professional every three years starting at age twenty and every year starting at age forty.

- Get a mammogram every one to two years starting at age forty and every year starting at age fifty (consider starting mammograms earlier if there's a strong family history).

- Limit alcohol intake.

- Consider using the prescription drugs raloxifene or tamoxifen if your doctor says you're eligible.

- Consider genetic testing for the BRCA genes. Presence of the genes greatly increases your risk of breast cancer. If you are BRCA-positive you will have to heighten your vigilance.

- Lose weight if you're overweight (see weight control section of chapter 5).

- Boost your immune system with good sleep, prayer, meditation, or social and community connectedness (chapter 5).

- Eat a healthy diet and exercise (see diet and exercise sections of chapter 5). Increasing your intake of soy-based foods may be the best dietary intervention for preventing breast cancer.

Breast cancer is a common disease, striking roughly 150,000 women and 1,000 men each year. About 44,000 die from the disease each year. Because more and more women are listening to the "mammogram message," the breast cancer survival rate in this country has improved over the past two and a half decades, from 74.5 percent in 1973 to 85.3 percent today. We can thank early diagnosis for most of these lives saved.

Mammograms are the most common and effective method of detecting breast cancer while it's still treatable. Soon, special ultrasound and MRI devices will be even more accurate and reliable than mammography. But no matter how sophisticated these screenings become, none of them will actually *prevent* breast cancer.

There's still much we need to know about the disease before we are sure which preventions work. The estrogen-like drug tamoxifen shows some potential, with trials suggesting a 50 percent reduction of new cancers. Drugs similar to tamoxifen, such as raloxifene, may give similar results. Unfortunately, both drugs are associated with an increased risk of blood clots and both can worsen menopausal symptoms such as hot flashes. The other preventive interventions are less studied but no less important.

Prostate Cancer Risk Factors

- Increasing age
- African-American heritage
- Family history, especially in a father or brother
- Diets high in saturated fat or red meat
- Cigarette smoking

Prostate Cancer Preventive Interventions

- Get a PSA (prostate specific antigen) blood test (free and total PSA levels) and a digital rectal exam every year starting at age forty. Improvements in PSA testing are being considered, including PSA density (comparing PSA level to size of prostate) and PSA velocity (tracking rise in PSA over time).
- Don't smoke!
- Avoid secondhand smoke.
- Limit alcohol intake.
- Boost your immune system with good sleep, prayer, meditation, social and community connectedness (chapter 5).
- Eat a healthy diet and exercise (see diet and exercise sections of chapter 5). Soy-based foods, tomato products, and selenium supplements show the most promise in prostate cancer prevention. Beef is the most potent prostate cancer–producing food known and should be avoided.
- Report any symptoms to your doctor that may be a sign of prostate enlargement such as more frequent urination, urinary dribbling, incontinence, slow or weak urine stream, or pain or burning with urination. All of these symptoms have causes other than cancer as well, and it will be up to your doctor to make the proper diagnosis.

Diabetes

Diabetes contributes to 169,000 deaths each year, many classified as heart disease or stroke. Diabetes normally refers to diabetes mellitus, two distinct diseases that involve either a shutdown in the production of the hormone insulin (in Type I diabetes), or a change in the body's ability to utilize insulin (Type II). Adult-onset (Type II) diabetes is about ten times more common then insulin-dependent (Type I or child-onset) diabetes; both can cause similar long-term complications such as blindness, kidney failure, heart disease, impotence, increased susceptibility to infection, peripheral nerve damage, and even arthritis.

Diabetes Risk Factors

- Family history (especially for Type II diabetes)
- Obesity (especially a large waist)
- Sedentary lifestyle
- African-American, Asian-American, Hispanic-American, Native American, or Pacific Island heritage
- Increasing age
- Fasting blood sugar level over 115. We start to watch closely when the fasting sugar level climbs over 100.
- Elevated glycated hemoglobin A1c. The test for this condition detects how much sugar is attached to the blood cells, an indicator of blood sugar levels over the past three months. High levels indicate blood sugar levels that are poorly controlled.
- Having diabetes while pregnant
- Delivering a baby over nine pounds

Diabetes Preventive Interventions

- Lose weight (if you're overweight, and especially if you have a large waist).
- Get a fasting blood sugar test every three years starting at age forty-five. Start getting tested at age twenty if you are obese or have a family history of diabetes.
- Eat a healthy diet and exercise (see diet and exercise sections of chapter 5). Exercise improves insulin sensitivity, which is decreased in both types of diabetes. Exercise is both a treatment and a preventive activity for Type II diabetes. Special attention should be paid to the diet. Many people with Type II diabetes improve their insulin sensitivity by consuming a diet that is higher in protein and lower in carbohydrates.

If You Have Diabetes

- Keep a tight control over fasting blood sugar. The closer the glucose level is to normal, the less likely secondary complications of diabetes will appear. For insulin-dependent diabetics, this may mean glucose testing and insulin shots four times daily.

- Aggressively control risk factors for heart disease (see above). Diabetes is a major risk factor for artery blockage, so control of cholesterol, blood pressure, and smoking is even more important in the diabetic patient. Blood pressure should definitely be kept below 130/85.

- Inspect legs and feet daily, looking especially for cuts and foot ulcers. With a decrease in sensation from nerve damage, and a decrease in the blood flow to the feet from the diabetes, painless ulcers can develop in the feet and legs. Caught early, they can be easily treated. Left untreated, amputation of the foot or leg may result. Amputations are about one hundred times more common in diabetic patients than in the general population.

- Get annual eye exams. Diabetes can lead to a host of eye problems and is a leading cause of blindness. Early detection of eye diseases can save your vision.

- Avoid infections. Yearly flu shots are a must, as is the pneumococcal vaccine (to help prevent certain forms of pneumonia).

- Limit alcohol consumption.

- Get a fasting cholesterol profile annually.

- Get a urinalysis for protein to detect kidney disease at every doctor visit. If protein is not found, test for microalbumin, a more sensitive measure of early kidney failure.

Osteoarthritis

The way to prevent and treat this condition is to do almost the exact opposite of what people are currently doing. Most of the 35 million people suffering from osteoarthritis take anti-inflammatory medications such as ibuprofen, aspirin, or about fifteen different prescription drugs that have the same mechanism of action. Once taking the pain medication, most patients continue to do the very things that resulted in the disease in the first place. Remember that the body experiences pain for a reason—it's a warning sign to change what you're doing. It just doesn't make sense to cover up this warning sign and continue to damage your joints. Glucosamine and chondroitin taken in combination help improve joint health. Find out all you need to know about these supplements at www.drtheo.com.

Osteoarthritis Risk Factors

- Family history (especially if the family member is affected in four or more joints, or if the fingers are involved)
- Congenital (present at birth) joint malalignment such as hip dysplasia
- Obesity (women in the top 20 percent of body weight are eight times more likely to develop knee osteoarthritis)
- Elevated levels of uric acid (a waste product that can lead to gout) and ferritin (stored iron)
- Joint injuries (especially ligament or cartilage tears and fractures that cross into a joint)
- High-risk sports (such as skiing, "X-games," football, soccer, basketball, volleyball, martial arts)
- Poor biomechanics (improper lifting techniques, abnormal gait, or joint movement patterns)
- Joint hypermobility (a loose or unstable joint)
- Surgical removal of joint cartilage (especially the meniscus cartilage in the knee)
- Manual labor occupations
- Low levels of vitamins B_6, B_{12}, folate, and vitamin D

Osteoarthritis Preventive Interventions

- Injury prevention—choose lower risk sports.
- Ensure proper recovery if injured (including formal physical therapy, if indicated).
- Lose weight, if overweight, and maintain ideal weight (see chapter 5).
- Get your blood checked for levels of uric acid and iron. If elevated, treat. Check for levels of vitamins B_{12} and D, and the mineral manganese. Supplement if levels are low.
- Eat a healthy diet (see chapter 5). It is especially important to eat a wide variety of fruits and vegetables.

- Perform regular, low-impact activities such as biking, weightlifting, swimming, and walking.
- Consider using glucosamine and chondroitin supplements. Chondroitin especially has been proven to reduce breakdown in joint cartilage with long-term use.
- Consider other supplements. Nutrients known to benefit joint health include vitamins B_6, B_{12}, folate, C, and D and the minerals boron and manganese. Antioxidants (see above) are also beneficial. For signs of inflammation (swelling, warmth, pain), omega-3 fatty acids (from flax oil) and GLA (from borage oil) have shown clinical improvement in human trials.
- Optimize your biomechanics. Poor biomechanics may be the biggest contributor to the development of osteoarthritis. Biomechanics refers to the way the body moves and distributes or absorbs force. When we lift something off the ground, for instance, bending the knees allows the force of the lift to be distributed throughout the body. Lifting with the knees straight causes most of the force to be concentrated in the lower back. It's no surprise that people with poor lifting technique develop back pain and osteoarthritis in their lower lumbar spine. Get a biomechanical exam by a sports medicine specialist or osteopathic physician.

Osteoporosis

Osteoporosis literally means "porous bones" and refers to loss of bone mineral content to the point where getting a fracture become much more likely. The death rate from osteoporosis, which affects 28 million people and causes 1.5 million fractures and 50,000 deaths a year, now exceeds that of breast cancer and continues to climb. Along with osteoarthritis, osteoporosis is what causes older people to "feel" old and frail. Unfortunately about 80 percent of the people with this condition do not know they are affected. There are no symptoms until a fracture occurs. The good news is that this condition is almost completely preventable if intervention is instituted early.

Osteoporosis Risk Factors

- Female (men are not immune; 20 percent of cases are in men)
- Thin or small frame (though you can't detect bone density by someone's appearance)

- Increasing age
- Early menopause
- Low levels of estrogen or testosterone
- Family history of menopause
- Caucasian or Asian heritage
- Sedentary lifestyle, especially lack of weight-bearing or strength-training activities
- Low calcium intake, lactose intolerance, eating disorders, chronic gastrointestinal malabsorption, inflammatory bowel disease, or stomach removal
- Low vitamin D levels
- Cigarette smoking
- Medical conditions including diabetes, liver or kidney disease, hyperthyroidism, or Cushing's syndrome (excess production of cortisol by the adrenal glands)
- Excessive alcohol, caffeine, or sodium intake
- Prolonged use of diuretics, laxatives, anticonvulsants (phenytoin, barbiturate), corticosteroids, anticoagulants (heparin, warfarin), some cholesterol-lowering agents (cholestyramine, colestipol), or excess thyroid hormone replacement

Osteoporosis Preventive Interventions

- Know your bone density. Bone loss can't be felt unless there's a fracture. Get a bone mineral density study when you're approaching menopause. Repeat the test every one to five years depending on the results.
- Get adequate calcium and magnesium (see supplement section in chapter 5 for exact dosage).
- Get the recommended daily value (400 IU) for vitamin D from a multivitamin, other supplements, or four servings of dairy per day. If you're over sixty-five, get 600 IU of vitamin D a day, unless a blood level of vitamin D shows that you need more or less vitamin D by supplement.
- Increase your intake of soy-based foods and consider supplemental soy isoflavones.
- Consider estrogen/progesterone replacement at menopause (women).

- Consider testosterone replacement (men and women) if low testosterone levels are suggested by symptoms (low libido) and documented by blood testing (for free and total testosterone level).
- Don't smoke!
- Limit caffeine intake.
- Eat a healthy diet and exercise (see diet and exercise sections of chapter 5). Weightlifting is one of the most potent preventive agents for osteoporosis.

Memory Loss

We've seen memory loss occur with age so often that most of us believe that age and memory loss go hand in hand. Several high-profile studies, however, suggest that memory loss may be preventable, and demonstrate the tremendous benefits of nutrition, exercise, social support, sleep, and community involvement. Conversely, unhealthy habits in any of these areas will, over time, contribute to memory loss in our later years.

The research into memory loss is ongoing, and may reveal more risk factors and preventions in coming years. But even if it turns out that none of these risk factors or preventions will affect your memory, they all will affect other parts of your health.

Memory Loss Risk Factors
- Increasing age
- Sedentary lifestyle
- Stress and high blood pressure
- Depression
- B vitamin deficiency
- Lack of "mental exercise"

Memory Loss Interventions
- Multivitamins, especially those with high levels of vitamin C and E
- Minerals, especially magnesium, zinc, and selenium
- Coenzyme Q-10
- Omega-3 and omega-6 essential fatty acids (found in seeds, certain fish, and in supplemental form)

- DMAE (dimethylamine ethanol)
- Acetyl L-carnitine
- DHEA (dehydroepiandrosterone)
- Lecithin
- Phosphatidylserine
- Ginko biloba
- Siberian ginseng
- Exercise, especially aerobic exercise
- Stress reduction
- Depression treatments, including therapy, medication, and social-community connectedness
- Exercise for the mind, such as crossword puzzles, learning a new language, or taking classes that require intensive memorization and recall
- Hormone replacement. We don't know the exact mechanism, but there seems to be a significantly lower rate of dementia in women using estrogen alone or with progesterone after menopause. We predict that men at high risk for Alzheimer's, cardiovascular disease, and perhaps even osteoporosis will someday use low-dose estrogen, or one of the "designer" estrogens, as a treatment.
- Long-term use of anti-inflammatory medications such as aspirin or ibuprofen may also be beneficial in preventing Alzheimer's. Unfortunately, long-term use of anti-inflammatory drugs can cause bleeding, liver, kidney damage, and medication interactions that lead to over 16,000 deaths per year.
- The new COX-2 inhibitors, anti-inflammatory medications with a lower side effect profile, are currently being evaluated for their prevention potential. These may be a breakthrough intervention for Alzheimer's since they are much safer than typical anti-inflammatory medications.
- B-complex vitamins look promising. It's alarming to see how many older folks are deficient in the B-complex vitamins. Vitamin B_{12} deficiency is the biggest culprit. Tens of thousands of people over sixty-five have low B_{12} levels. Unfortunately, most physicians recognize this deficiency in its latter stages when the patient's red blood cells have become enlarged and anemia is detected with a routine blood test. The deficiency must be recognized much sooner, before psychological changes have a chance to manifest.

~ Appendix D ~
Dietary Supplements
to Avoid

Keep in mind that anything powerful enough to change the body is powerful enough to harm the body in some way. Don't fall into the trap of thinking that if something is natural, it's automatically safe and good for you. Arsenic, mercury, hemlock, lead, cobra venom, uranium, and great white sharks are 100 percent natural, but you'd be better off keeping away from them. Many plant products, sold as fresh herbs and as manufactured supplements, can also cause harm. A third of the pharmaceutical products on the market are derived directly from plants and are considered drugs.

Here's a selected list of some complementary and alternative treatments you should approach with caution, if at all:

Colloidal minerals. Touted by "quacks" to be the "missing link" that cures and prevents almost everything, these products can be downright dangerous. Colloids are a mixture of solid substances suspended (but not dissolved) into a liquid. These products are generally little more than some dirt shaken into water, with added flavoring and coloring. Colloidal mineral products should be avoided. Most contain toxic heavy metals such as lead, arsenic, and mercury in addition to some radioactive materials not known to have any benefit for human health. We are surprised the FDA allows these products to be sold.

The manufacturers and distributors of these products correctly note that trace mineral dietary deficiencies can lead to health problems. These minerals, however, can be provided by safe, pure supplements as we discuss in chapter 5.

5-HTP (5-hydroxy-L-tryptophan). 5-HTP is a compound purported to help with depression, sleep, and weight loss. Beware—it may be dangerous, even deadly. The cousin of 5-HTP, L-tryptophan, was banned several years ago by the FDA after it was associated with dozens of deaths and thousands of sick people. A contaminant called Peak X was found in some L-tryptophan products. Peak X, by itself or with other contaminants, appears to be linked with a condition called EMS (eosinophilia-myalgia syndrome).

Recent independent testing by researchers at the Mayo Clinic found that six products from six different companies containing 5-HTP all contained Peak X, whether the 5-HTP was from natural or artificial sources. Though the Peak X level in the 5-HTP products was lower than that in the L-tryptophan products, the large doses of 5-HTP recommended by at least one book would appear to expose people to similar (and dangerous) amounts of Peak X. In addition, 5-HTP is not normally found in the bloodstream, and no one knows what will happen to people who consume this supplement on a long-term basis. Even some 5-HTP researchers scoff at the use of this product by the public. We feel it is irresponsible to recommend 5-HTP product at this time.

Aconite or "bushi." This herb isn't too widely used here, and hopefully it never will be. It's been tied to several poisonings in China after the subjects took it for rheumatic complaints, headaches, or general pain relief.

N-acetyl glucosamine (NAG). Unlike its cousins glucosamine HCL and sulfate, NAG is not very effective for helping joints and stimulating cartilage. Don't waste your money on products containing this substance.

Poke root. A slow emetic and purgative, poke root is also used in chronic rheumatic disease. Overdoses may produce vomiting, convulsions, and death. Avoid.

Comfrey. Even though it's not usually taken internally, comfrey— usually used for cuts, bruises, and ulcers—is very dangerous. The toxins in this plant have been linked to liver damage and death.

Borage. Research isn't complete, but it looks like this herb may pack a host of toxins that affect the liver. It may even contain carcinogens. Some people recommend it for coughs or as a mood booster, but there are plenty of safe and natural alternatives to this potentially danger-ous herb. Don't confuse borage plant parts with borage oil. The bor-age oil supplements are considered to be safe.

Ephedra (ephedrine). Ephedrine is a stimulant with a molecular structure and function similar to amphetamine. This drug is an ingre-dient in diet pills, illicit recreational drugs, and some legitimate over-the-counter decongestants. Ephedrine has been associated with the following: heart attack and stroke, palpitations, paranoid psychosis, convulsions, depression, coma, vomiting, hypertension, and respira-tory depression.

Blue cohosh. Blue cohosh has been used to relieve menstrual cramps. It contains caulosaponin, a blood vessel constrictor that can also stim-ulate uterine contractions and induce childbirth. Don't confuse with black cohosh, a safer herb that can be helpful for relieving symptoms of menopause.

Chaparral. Often held out as a magic bullet for people with arthritis, cancer, and colds, this herb can cause severe hepatitis, leading to liver failure.

Germander. Used to cure digestive problems and fever, germander contains a powerful stimulant that can cause heart problems in some people.

Skullcap. Used as a tranquilizer, this drug can cause serious liver dam-age, confusion, and even convulsions.

Kombucha tea. Used for a wide range of problems, from AIDS to acne, this herb has been linked to liver problems, intestinal problems, and even deaths.

Lobelia. Some people use lobelia as a pick-me-up. Some of these users have experienced rapid heartbeat. Several comas and deaths have been tied to this herb.

Broom. Here's another potent drug that may cause the same prob-lems quack herbalists say it solves. Broom is taken for heart problems, but may slow a subject's heart rhythms. Even if it doesn't, the level of toxic alkaloids it contains is unacceptable.

Pennyroyal. The list of problems linked to pennyroyal includes liver damage, convulsions, miscarriages, and comas. Several deaths have also been reported. Don't go near this "remedy" for gastric problems.

Sassafras. This herb, once widely used in cooking, was banned after it was discovered to cause cancer. Some people still use it as a stimulant.

Wormwood. This herb was once used to make absinthe; some now say it's good for digestion. Those people usually don't mention that it can cause convulsions, loss of consciousness, and hallucinations.

Even if you don't have an immediate negative reaction to these herbs, long-term use can cause permanent damage. They all may react negatively with over-the-counter and prescription medication, which can amplify their effects. The best way to avoid those interactions is to avoid these "remedies." But since new herbs are being adopted for medicinal use all the time, this list is incomplete. That's why we have to say again, always let your doctor know if you are taking any herbal remedies. Bring them with you, or if you can't, use the form in appendix A. Fortunately, doctors are learning more and more about herbs, and new reference texts have made it easy for your doctor to screen for potential interactions.

~

Selected Bibliography

Acs, Gregory, and John Sabelhaus. "Trends in Out-of-Pocket Spending on Health Care, 1980–1992." *Monthly Labor Review*, December 1995, 35–45.

American Academy of Pediatrics Committee on Children with Disabilities. "Managed Care and Children with Special Health Care Needs: A Subject Review." *Pediatrics* 102, no. 3 (1998): 657–60.

American Journal of Managed Care. "Special Report: Looking Beyond the Formulary Budget." 1997.

Anders, George. *Health against Wealth: HMOs and the Breakdown of Medical Trust.* Boston: Houghton Mifflin, 1996.

Bates, Barbara, M.D. *A Guide to Physical Examination and History Taking.* 5th ed. Philadelphia: J. B. Lippincott, 1991.

Blostin, Allan P., and Jordan N. Pfunter. "Employee Medical Care Contributions on the Rise." *Compensation and Working Conditions* 3, no. 1 (1998).

Bodenheimer, Thomas, M.D., and Kip Sullivan, J.D. "How Large Employers Are Shaping the Health Care Marketplace." *Health Policy Report* 338, no. 14 (1998): 1003–8.

Bucci, Michael, and Robert Grant. "Employer-Sponsored Health Insurance: What's Offered; What's Chosen." *Monthly Labor Review*, October 1995, 38–44.

Castro, Janice. *The American Way of Health: How Medicine Is Changing and What It Means to You.* Boston: Little Brown, 1994.

Cheney, Karen. "How to Be a Managed Care Winner." *Money*, July 1997, 122–31.

Columbia University College of Physicians and Surgeons. *Complete Guide to Early Child Care.* New York: Crown, 1990.

Davidoff, Frank, M.D. "Medicine and Commerce—1. Is Managed Care a 'Monstrous Hybrid?'" *Annals of Internal Medicine* 128, no. 6 (1998): 496–99.

Emanuel, Ezekiel, M.D., and Nancy Neveloff Dubler, L.L.B. "Preserving the Physician-Patient Relationship in the Era of Managed Care." *Journal of the American Medical Association* 273, no. 4 (1995): 323–29.

Enzmann, Dieter R. *Surviving in Health Care*. St. Louis: Mosby, 1997.

Finkelstein, Katherine Eban. "The Sick Business." *New Republic*, December 29, 1997, 23–27.

Gorman, Christine. "Playing the HMO Game." *Time*, July 13, 1998, 22–29.

Gresenz, Carole Roan, Ph.D., Xiofeng Liu, M.D., M.S., and Roland Sturum, Ph.D. "Managed Care Behavioral Health Services for Children under Carve-Out Contracts." *Psychiatric Services* 49, no. 8 (1998): 1054–1058.

Griffith, H. Winter, M.D. *The Complete Guide to Symptoms, Illness, and Surgery*. 3rd ed. New York: The Body Press/Perigee, 1995.

Grüninger, V. J. "Patient Education: An Example of One-to-One Communication." *Journal of Human Hypertension* 9 (1995): 15–25.

Hall, Mark A., J.D., and Robert A. Berenson, M.D. "Ethical Practices in Managed Care: A Dose of Realism." *Annals of Internal Medicine* 128, no. 5 (1998): 395–402.

Heagarty, Margaret C., M.D., and William J. Moss, M.D., M.P.H. *Pediatrics*. Philadelphia: Lippincott-Raven, 1997.

Health Care Advisory Board. "The Impact of Managed Care on the Health Care Industry." 1997.

———. "Managed Care Project #3: Insurer-Denied Days: Benchmarks, Appeal Process, and Strategies for Reduction." 1998.

Hymowitz, Carol. "Psychotherapy Patients Pay a Price for Privacy." *Wall Street Journal*, January 22, 1998.

Kalish, Bradley. "PPOs Deliver What HMOs Don't." *Modern Healthcare*, April 20, 1996.

Kaplan, Sherrie H., Ph.D., M.P.H., Barbara Gandek, M.S., Sheldon Greenfield, M.D., William Rogers, Ph.D., and John E. Ware, Ph.D. "Patient and Visit Characteristics Related to Physicians' Decision-Making Style." *Medical Care* 33, no. 12 (1995): 1176–87.

Kerr, Eve A., M.D., M.P.H., et al. "Primary Care Physicians' Satisfaction with Quality of Care in California Capitated Medical Groups." *Journal of the American Medical Association* 278, no. 4 (1997): 308–12.

Kuttner, Robert. "Must Good HMOs Go Bad? The Commercialization of Prepaid Group Health Care." *New England Journal of Medicine* 338, no. 21 (1998): 1558–63.

———. "Must Good HMOs Go Bad? The Search for Checks and Balances." *New England Journal of Medicine* 338, no. 22 (1998): 1635–39.

Lawrence, Jean. "They're Coaching Your Patients on What to Demand from You." *Managed Care*, June 1997, 42–47.

Lee, Jason S. "Managed Health Care: A Primer." Congressional Research Service, 1997.

Leslie, Frederikson. "Exploring Information Exchange in Consultation: The Patients' View of Performance and Outcomes." *Patient Education and Counseling* 25 (1995): 237–46.

Leslie, Lauren K., M.D. "Child Health Care in Changing Times." *Pediatrics* 101, no. 4 (1998): 746–52.

Lipkin, Mack Jr., Samuel M. Putnam, and Aaron Lazare, eds. *The Medical Interview*. New York: Springer-Verlag, 1995.

Marquis, Julie. "Doctors Who Lose Patience." *Los Angeles Times*, March 3, 1999, A1.

McCann, S., and J. Weinman. "Empowering the Patient in the Consultation: A Pilot Study." *Patient Education and Counseling* 27 (1996): 227–34.

Mechanic, David, Ph.D., and Mark Schlesinger, Ph.D. "The Impact of Managed Care on Patient's Trust in Medical Care and Their Physicians." *Journal of the American Medical Association* 275, no. 21 (1996): 1693–97.

Meckler, Laura. "HMO Debate Shifts to What Is 'Medically Necessary.'" Associated Press, March 3, 1999.

Millenson, Michael. *Demanding Medical Excellence: Doctors and Accountability in the Information Age*. Chicago: University of Chicago Press, 1997.

Moore, J.D., Jr. "Doctors against Profits (Except Their Own)." *Wall Street Journal*, December 17, 1997.

Nixon, J. Peter. "Health Care Reform: A Labor Perspective." In *Health Care Reform in the Nineties*, edited by Pauline Vaillancourt Rosenau. Thousand Oaks, CA: Sage, 1994.

Offson, Mark, M.D., M.P.H., Steven C. Marcus, Ph.D., and Harold Alan Pincus, M.D. "Trends in Office-Based Psychiatric Practice." *American Journal of Psychiatry* 156, no. 3 (1999): 451–57.

Ong, L. M. L., J. C. J. M. de Haes, A. M. Hoos, and F. B. Lammes. "Doctor-Patient Communication: A Review of the Literature." *Social Science and Medicine* 40, no. 7 (1995): 903–18.

Pollock, Ellen Joan. "In Buyer's Market, Fee Negotiations Are Delicate Dance." *Wall Street Journal*, January 22, 1998.

Reed, Susan E. "Miss Treatment." *New Republic*, December 29, 1997, 20–23.

Reno, Robert. "Fibbing to the HMOs Just What the Doctor Ordered." *Minneapolis Star Tribune*, November 19, 1998, 21A.

Reynolds, Richard, M.D., and John Stone, M.D., eds. *On Doctoring*. Revised and expanded ed. New York: Simon & Schuster, 1995.

Roter, Debra L., and Judith A. Hall. *Doctors Talking with Patients/Patients Talking with Doctors*. Westport, CT: Auburn House, 1992.

Ryer, Jeanne C. *HealthNet: Your Essential Resource for the Most Up-to-Date Medical Information Online*. New York: John Wiley & Sons, 1997.

Spragins, Ellyn. *Choosing and Using an HMO*. New York: Bloomberg, 1997.

————. "When Your HMO Says No." *Newsweek*, July 28, 1997, 73.

Starr, Paul. *The Social Transformation of American Medicine*. New York: Basic Books, 1982.

Stoline, Anne M., M.D., and Jonathan P. Weiner, Ph.D. *The New Medical Marketplace: A Physician's Guide to the Health Care System in the 1990s*. Baltimore: Johns Hopkins University Press, 1993.

Stroul, Beth A., Sheila A. Pires, Mary I. Armstrong, and Judith C. Meyers. "The Impact of Managed Care on Mental Health Services for Children and Their Families." *The Future of Children* 8, no. 2 (1998): 119–33.

Taylor, Roger, and Leeba Lessin. "Restructuring the Health Care Delivery System in the United States." *Journal of Health Care Finance* 22, no. 4 (1996): 33–60.

Terry, Ken. "No Cause Terminations: Will They Go Up in Flames?" *Medical Economics*, February 1998, 22–29.

USA Today. "Doctors Fudge Truth to Avoid HMO Care Denials." November 11, 1998.

U.S. Department of Labor, Office of the Chief Economist. "A Look at Employers' Costs of Providing Health Insurance." Washington, D.C.: 1996.

U.S. News & World Report, Editors of. *America's Best Hospitals*. New York: John Wiley & Sons, 1996.

Yale University School of Medicine, Faculty Members at the. *The Patient's Guide to Medical Tests*. Boston: Houghton Mifflin, 1997.

Index